RUNNING IN PLACE

THE DEVOLUTION REVOLUTION

A series of Century Foundation Reports that analyzes the impact of the widespread shift of government responsibilities from the national to the state and local level.

OTHER REPORTS IN THE SERIES INCLUDE:

HAZARDOUS CROSSCURRENTS: Confronting Inequality in an Era of Devolution by **John D. Donahue**

MEDICAID AND THE STATES by **Paul Offner**

CAN THE STATES AFFORD DEVOLUTION? The Fiscal Implications of Shifting Federal Responsibilities to State and Local Governments by **Harold A. Hovey**

Running in Place

How the Medicaid Model Falls Short, and What to Do About It

Eliot Fishman

A CENTURY FOUNDATION REPORT

The Century Foundation Press • New York

Cataloging in Publication Data

Fishman, Eliot
 Running in place : how the Medicaid model falls short, and what to do about it / Eliot Fishman.
  p. cm. -- (The devolution revolution)
 "A Century Foundation report."
 Includes bibliographical references and index.
  ISBN 0-87078-477-3 (alk. paper)
 1. Medicaid. 2. Medical Policy--United States
  [DNLM: 1. Medicaid--organization & administration. 2. Medicaid--economics. 3. Models, Economic--United States. 4. State.Government--United States. W 250 AA1 F537r 2002] I. Title: How the Medicaid model falls short, and what to do about it. II. Title. III. Series.
RA412.4 .F55 2002
368.4'2'00973--dc21   2002007780

Cover design and illustration: Claude Goodwin
Manufactured in the United States of America.

49859928

FOREWORD

R obert Putnam's *Making Democracy Work: Civic Traditions in Modern Italy* was one of the most important works of social science of the late twentieth century. The result of twenty-five years of study, it explored, among other things, a range of possible explanations for the dramatically differing performances of the regional government structures put in place in Italy beginning in 1970. Putnam drew many important conclusions from his study, including the widely cited observation that significant differences in civic culture, some nearly a thousand years in the making, appear to be highly correlated with the relative success or failure of these experiments in subnational government.

While there have been numerous attempts to apply Putnam's analytical approach to other parts of the world, I know of no evidence that it was part of the debate about just what would happen if substantial national responsibilities were "devolved" to the fifty states. Devolution, in general, is seen as a good thing to implement wherever possible. This, despite (or maybe because of) the fact that the existing diversity among the states, both real and imaginary, is more celebrated than studied. We accept as tolerable the existing great divergence in wealth, income, and the provision of public services among the several states. But certainly it is no cause for jubilation that infant mortality ranges from 10.5 per 1,000 live births in Mississippi to 5.2 in Massachusetts. Nor can the wide gulf between the highest-performing states in elementary and secondary education and the bottom tier be the result of an immutable preference for diversity.

Now, because of the movement in recent decades to give the states a larger role in such programs as Medicaid, welfare, and housing, these questions have taken on a new importance. For the one sure consequence of devolution is that it will result in a wider range of administrative arrangements, means of intervention, and levels of assistance for citizens affected by these programs. Given this, the Trustees of The Century Foundation decided that serious research and analysis on the impact of devolution could be of real value to policymakers and the public.

This volume in our series on devolution is especially timely. In it, Eliot Fishman, a senior research associate at the Institute for Medicare Practice at Mount Sinai School of Medicine, analyzes the various means-tested health insurance initiatives instituted since the 1960s. He finds that, although there have been successes, on the whole these programs never have come close to fulfilling the high expectations they raised about enrollment and access. Today, despite the creation of various state-run programs targeted at the poor, millions of Americans, including many of the poorest and most vulnerable, go without health insurance.

The State Children's Health Insurance Program, known as CHIP, the most recent and the most touted of these programs, has registered some apparently impressive gains in enrollment. But Fishman argues that these advances have made barely a dent at best in overall insurance rates for children because of a decline in private employer coverage. In addition, states facing budget shortfalls already have begun to cut back on their CHIP programs by capping spending and tightening eligibility requirements. These cutbacks—which could become more severe if our current fiscal crises deepen—threaten to erode previous gains in children's insurance coverage and may hinder the chances for states to qualify for the full possible amount of federal matching funds.

Without comprehensive health care reform, Fishman argues, increasing the effectiveness of existing state-run programs will require the federal government to assume more of the financial cost of these programs. More people would be covered if enrollment was automatic and eligibility verified retrospectively. Moreover, the appeal of such programs would increase if they were broadened to include working families having trouble finding affordable insurance, which would remove the stigma of any association with welfare.

Three other reports in this series have been published: *Hazardous Crosscurrents: Confronting Inequality in an Era of Devolution* by John D. Donahue, *Can the States Afford Devolution? The Fiscal Implications of Shifting Federal Responsibilities to State and Local Governments* by Harold A. Hovey, and *Medicaid and the States* by Paul Offner; another, looking at housing policy, is planned.

Fishman has highlighted the consequences of past policy choices and clarified those we shall face in the future. On behalf of the Trustees of The Century Foundation, I thank him for his work on this important and difficult issue.

RICHARD C. LEONE, *President*
The Century Foundation
July 2002

Contents

1

INTRODUCTION

On a typically hot August afternoon in Washington in 1997, President Bill Clinton signed a law creating the State Children's Health Insurance Program, known as CHIP. The program was a relatively small part of a massive budget bill, and Clinton signed it surrounded by American flags and congressional leaders, with a Marine band performing "God Bless America" on the White House balcony and a thousand people looking on. Still, Clinton made children's health coverage a major theme of a day in which he announced that "the sun is rising on America again." The program, he declared, would be the "largest expansion in health care for children since the Medicaid program 32 years ago." The White House predicted it would cut the number of uninsured children in half, from 10 million to 5 million, by sending money to the states to cover children in low-income families that earned too much money to qualify for Medicaid, a similar state-federal health insurance program. A *Washington Post* editorial by the sponsors of the legislation, Senators Ted Kennedy and Orrin Hatch, was even more effusive, declaring the program's creation to be "the most significant health reform since the enactment of Medicare and Medicaid in 1965, representing one of the most far-reaching steps the country has ever taken to help the nation's children." As they noted in a careful phrasing, "The funds allocated under the act are sufficient to give 5 million children the access they need for affordable health insurance."[1]

However many children those funds should have covered in principle, the results have been unimpressive so far. The most recent figures for child insurance coverage, from 2000, show that the number of uninsured children has dropped by only about 1 million. And the percentage receiving government coverage is actually slightly less than it was in 1997, meaning that all of this improvement was the result of the (formerly) strong economy rather than CHIP enrollment.[2] It was only more than three years after the law was signed that every state had a CHIP program up and running. And it was only after similar delays that the program started to enroll significant numbers of children—not close to the 5 million children envisioned in 1997 but exceeding 3 million (still few enough that many states would have been required to forfeit unspent federal CHIP funds until Congress gave them an extension in late 2000).

These figures are particularly disheartening when compared to Medicare's early performance. Medicare began full operations a year after Lyndon Johnson signed the program into existence in 1965. It achieved virtually universal coverage of the elderly in its first year, and that included the physician insurance program, which was and is a voluntary program for seniors. Medicare took a population with poor health coverage and covered that population in a year—period.

CHIP has been the most prominent of a series of proposals for incremental, de-centralized expansions of health coverage that have dominated health policy across the political spectrum since the failure of the Clinton health reform effort in 1994. The proposals have mostly fallen into a specific pattern: benefits targeted at the poor or near-poor, run by the states and paid for by both states and the federal government. And this is nothing new—with the obvious and important exception of Medicare (though inroads have been made into Medicare as well), a similar model has dominated public health insurance in the United States for more than forty years.

This "run by the states, targeted at the poor" structure is a perennially effective legislative sell. It has emerged as a leading contender in the two main contemporary debates in American health coverage policy—prescription drug benefits for the elderly and subsidized health insurance for the working poor. Federal matching funding for means-tested coverage by the states has become the mainstream Democratic proposal for expanded health coverage for the nonelderly uninsured. Al Gore proposed a major expansion of CHIP to parents of enrolled children during his 2000 presidential campaign, a proposal that continues to have strong support from Democrats in Congress. Ron Pollack, head of the major liberal health care lobby Families USA, has been trumpeting Medicaid and CHIP expansion as part of a joint health reform proposal with the American Hospital Association and the Health Insurance Association of America. And the Bush administration (and, previously, the Bush campaign) has consistently advocated a program of grants to states to offer means-tested prescription drug coverage for seniors as an "immediate helping hand" and as a provisional alternative to a broader Medicare prescription drug benefit, although this proposal initially met with significant skepticism from both parties in Congress.

To sum up, there is long-standing and continuing support in Washington for public health insurance on the "Medicaid model"— that is, targeted by income and operated by the states within federal guidelines. That model is central to the current American health care system, and it provides health coverage to tens of millions of vulnerable Americans. But it also consistently falls short of its main legislative objectives. Enrollment, access to health care, or both have been disappointing in many states. Many states cannot (or will not) enroll a substantial portion of those eligible under their own rules, and those rules themselves often exclude many who belong to the population ostensibly targeted by the federal authorizing legislation. These failures are most notable in the high proportion of the poor not eligible for or enrolled in Medicaid, by far the largest of the programs of this type; as we have seen, the same pathology has limited the much-hyped Children's Health Insurance Program as well. Furthermore, many physicians and mainstream health care plans do not participate in Medicaid, partly because payment to physicians and plans is often well below what they receive from Medicare and private payers.

While the political appeal of running health coverage through the states and targeting it at the poor is as strong as ever, the serious problems similar programs have encountered time and again have never entered the policy discussion. That absence was strikingly clear in the 2000 presidential debates. George Bush, following some Republicans in Congress, proposed to send money to the states to cover prescription drugs for the poor elderly, as a quick way to get coverage to those who need it most. He made much of the ease of fast implementation of the plan in both the first and second debates:

> I cannot let this go by—the old-style Washington politics of we're going to scare you in the voting booth. Under my plan, the man gets immediate help with prescription drugs. It's called immediate helping hand. Instead of squabbling and finger pointing, he gets immediate help.

> So what I want to do is I want to call upon Republicans and Democrats to forget all the arguing and finger pointing and come together and take care of our seniors with a pre-scription drug program that says we'll pay for the poor seniors, we'll help all seniors with prescription drugs. In the meantime, I think it's important to have what's called immediate helping hand, which is direct money to states so that seniors, poor seniors, don't have to choose between food and medicine.

But Bush was soon defending (later in the second debate) the long delays in implementation and enrollment in Texas for its CHIP program, precisely the same sort of state-run, federally mandated health program:

> Our CHIPS [sic] program got a late start because our gov-ernment meets only four months out of every two years, Mr. Vice President. May come for a shock for somebody who's been in Washington for so long, but actually limited government can work, in the second-largest state in the union. And therefore Congress passes the bill after our ses-sion in 1997 ended, we passed the enabling legislation in '99. . . . I signed a bill that puts CHIPS in place. The bill finally came out at the end of the '99 session. We're work-ing hard to sign up children.

Al Gore was in no position to point out this discrepancy, however. His own administration had strongly supported the passage of CHIP, and his own health reform proposals centered on a dramatic expansion of that underperforming state-run program, as he described in the same exchange in the second debate:

I'd like to see, eventually, in this country, some form of universal health care, but I'm not for a government-run system. . . . So I want to proceed carefully to cover more people. But I think that we should start by greatly expanding the so-called child health insurance, or CHIP program, to give health insurance to every single child in this country.

As Gore's statement makes clear, CHIP has political marketability going for it: it was and is a way to cover the uninsured without dramatically reducing the scope of private coverage, and without administering a new public program in Washington. But it has not moved us significantly closer to covering "every single child in this country." The American preference for targeting health reforms by income and running them through the states is all about ideology rather than effectiveness.

Like Gore, proponents in both parties of expansions of Medicaid-like programs are mostly sincere advocates of universal health insurance coverage of Americans through a combination of private and public coverage. This report shares that agenda, although it demonstrates that incremental expansions of the Medicaid model are unlikely to get us there.

In the following chapter, I will show how a series of similar programs have fallen short of their basic objectives, whether by not enrolling much of their target populations, not making eligible many of those in need, or giving those who are enrolled inadequate health coverage.

In Chapter 3, I explain what is causing state-run, means-tested programs to fall short so often. I lay out five underlying problems with the Medicaid model:

1. Working people and "welfare" programs do not mix;

2. The hassle of documenting income;

3. The political weakness of poor people's programs;

4. The irrelevance of health care in state elections;

5. The states with the most need have the least resources.

I also describe why the model is so popular with policymakers in Washington despite these problems. Washington likes Medicaid expansion both because it keeps bureaucracy in the states—and many in Washington do not consider state bureaucracies to be nearly as reprehensible as national ones—and because it does not affect the employment-based health coverage of most Americans.

In the final chapter of the report, I explore some politically plausible alternative structures for targeted health insurance. These directly address the problems laid out in Chapter 3 while trying to retain the features that give the Medicaid model its political popularity. The reforms include:

1. Changing the structure of means-tested health insurance programs to enroll people automatically and verify eligibility retrospectively;

2. Broadening the reach of state-administered programs to include portions of the middle class who cannot get health insurance;

3. Shifting more of the funding responsibility for means-tested health insurance programs to the federal government.

As of this writing, both a state-run prescription drug benefit and a Medicaid/CHIP expansion stand a fair chance of becoming law. Yet there is also a better than fair chance that, should either pass, the legislation will achieve little in the short term and will fall short of its goals in the long term. As we will see in the next chapter, underenrollment, underfunding, and operational problems have plagued a series of state-federal health insurance programs. This pattern began with the Kerr-Mills program for the elderly that preceded Medicare in the early sixties, and it has continued in Medicaid and Medicaid-related programs, the Children's Health Insurance Program, and, tellingly, in a variety of state-initiated "drug assistance" programs aimed at helping the elderly pay for prescriptions and health insurance programs. These kinds of programs are relatively easy to pass in Washington, but typically they do not work well. We can do better.

2

STATE-RUN AND MEANS-TESTED:
A BRIEF SUMMARY OF A
LONG HISTORY OF PROBLEMS

States operate a number of means-tested health insurance programs, most of them with federal mandates and matching funding.
Health insurance programs on the Medicaid model—means-tested,
and state-administered within federal guidelines—have played a
central role in the American health system since 1960. Initiatives following this model now include the original Medicaid program, the
large Medicaid expansions beginning in the late 1980s, the
"Medicare Buy-in" (Qualified Medicare Beneficiary/Specified Low-
Income Medicare Beneficiary, or QMB/SLMB) program, and the
State Children's Health Insurance Program (CHIP). Many states
also operate one or more means-tested health programs without
federal matching funds (or by drawing on a loose federal block
grant).

Some of these programs are clear success stories: some states
have enrolled even more people into their health programs than
surveys had shown to be eligible, and other states have aggressively expanded coverage levels, eligibility levels, and/or participation of
mainstream providers in one or more health programs without dramatic increases in expenditures. Some states have pioneered efforts
to give health coverage to uninsured adults or prescription drug

coverage to seniors, issues the federal government has been unable to deal with despite repeated attempts and widespread public support.

Yet formal eligibility levels, enrollment, and access to mainstream physician offices have often been disappointing in many states. Underenrollment has even been a problem—indeed, a particularly large problem—in those state-initiated programs to help the elderly pay for prescription drugs.

The contrast with Medicare, as noted in the previous chapter, is nearly total. Medicare Part B, covering physician and other outpatient expenses, was and is a voluntary program. Yet it enrolled 93 percent of the nation's senior citizens—17.7 million people—in its first year.[1] Both enrollment levels and access to physicians have been an overwhelming success story in Medicare, whereas one or both have been perennial problems in the state-federal programs, as the history recounted below will show.

1960–1965: Kerr-Mills

Problems of underenrollment and underfinancing were especially severe in the Kerr-Mills program, a short-lived predecessor of both Medicare and Medicaid in the early 1960s. By 1960, renewed political pressure for national health insurance for the elderly had been building for two years.[2] The Kerr-Mills bill of that year was a rearguard effort by conservative Democrats and Republicans to do something about that pressure without substantially increasing the scope of national government. It provided medical care to the indigent elderly using what is now Medicaid's structure: federal standards would set a comprehensive package of benefits for the elderly poor (or those elderly whose medical expenses rendered them effectively poor), while the specific eligibility guidelines, coverage features, and provider reimbursement levels would be set by the states. States would pay for the program with a federal match ranging from 50 to 80 percent, depending on state income levels.

Kerr-Mills was widely regarded as a near total disappointment. In its five years of existence (before it was replaced by Medicare), only five states established substantial programs. They received almost 90 percent of the total funds in 1963, and they still spent 70 percent of the national total (and received more than 60 percent of the federal matching funding) in 1965.[3] These states had all been funding their own health insurance programs for the poor elderly before 1960, so Kerr-Mills amounted to a federal grant to supplement their existing programs. Eighteen states had no program in place at all by 1964, and most of the states never set serious coverage and enrollment levels.

1965–Present: Medicaid

In 1965, at the same time that Medicare largely supplanted the Kerr-Mills program for the elderly, Kerr-Mills was expanded into the Medicaid program, both to continue to offer non-Medicare health benefits (such as long-term care and drug coverage) to the poorest elderly and to provide health care coverage for two other poor populations—single-parent families and the disabled. These three populations were already eligible in principle for cash welfare payments, and until the late 1980s Medicaid enrollment was typically an adjunct of welfare enrollment. The states had an option to make significant exceptions to the welfare-Medicaid connection: to enroll families poor enough for welfare (welfare for single parents was also known as AFDC) but with two parents (those with "Ribicoff children," after an amendment sponsored by Senator Abraham Ribicoff), or those whose incomes were above welfare levels but whose medical expenses effectively brought them below the threshold ("medically needy"). Finally, a provision of the legislation required states to move toward comprehensive medical coverage of Medicaid enrollees and "liberalized eligibility" for Medicaid. To sum up, the states were mandated to enroll their welfare population in Medicaid, and they had a substantial degree of latitude to set reimbursement rates and to expand eligibility beyond welfare.

Medicaid was and is successful in important respects: enrollment grew quickly initially and is larger than ever today, and enrollees have consistently received more regular medical care than the uninsured through that time.[4] But cost concerns soon became central to Medicaid policy in many states, and these states made cost-cutting moves that blunted the program's impact. Most states stinted on payment rates to doctors (and most still do), and Medicaid recipients often continued to rely on the same charity care facilities that they had used before the program (and many often still do), in part because of those low payment rates.[5] For decades, many states did not take up the options to enroll Ribicoff children and the medically needy despite federal money to defray most of the expense. (This has changed—federal mandates have phased in required enrollment of all poor children since 1990, while now most states do cover the medically needy.) More recently, states have failed to enroll a significant minority of Medicaid-eligible, uninsured people, although much of this problem may be the result of more fundamental flaws in the program's structure rather than state policy.

The problems described here (and in more detail below) are serious—in many states, eligibility for Medicaid is set tightly, enrollment of those eligible is disappointing, and access to mainstream care for enrollees is hit-or-miss. Nevertheless, it is important to emphasize that Medicaid is very far from the flop that Kerr-Mills was. Most notably, despite the underenrollment problem, Medicaid covers a lot of people, now even more than Medicare. Although cost concerns have long headlined state Medicaid politics, they are usually tempered by important initiatives to extend Medicaid coverage. Almost all states spend substantial amounts of optional money on Medicaid—that is, they offer significant levels of coverage or enroll large numbers of people that federal law does not require. About two-thirds of Medicaid spending is not required by federal law, and almost half of all Medicaid spending is for people that states do not have to cover.[6] In the most important example, by the 1990s more than two-thirds of states covered people whose medical expenses are high enough effectively to impoverish them, even if their nominal incomes are higher than Medicaid maximum levels—the "medically needy" coverage option mentioned above. More recently, a small but significant group of states have expanded their Medicaid programs through federally approved waivers of statutory rules and "income disregards" (the way the Medicaid statute allows states to raise income limits for the program for parents) to enroll employed, uninsured parents and childless adults, populations that have been essentially ignored in federal legislation.

And even in the many states in which Medicaid has been a troubled program, the problems are largely not the fault of the state governments. While some of them stem from underfunding—itself a result of the low priority on health spending in the politics of most states—there is a good deal more to it than that, as we will see in the next chapter. Some of these problems probably have to do with the inherent requirements of means testing and with the unfair burdens means-tested programs place on the poorest states.

Welfare Medicaid: 1965–1988

Medicaid's enactment coincided with a boom in enrollment in the preexisting welfare program for poor mothers and children—Aid to Families with Dependent Children (AFDC), which in turn drove unanticipated increases in Medicaid enrollment. Medicaid's rolls grew from 10 million people in 1967 to 24 million in 1976, largely paralleling similar growth in AFDC.[7] Medicaid's expenses grew even faster, as a result of rapid cost inflation in hospitals and nursing homes—from $3.5 billion to $14 billion.[8]

The states reacted to this growth by cutting back on coverage, reimbursement, and enrollment. States imposed a variety of limits on coverage for hospitalizations and physician office visits in the early 1970s, and these limits were especially draconian in the South. Levels of Medicaid reimbursement for primary care were held substantially lower than prevailing rates in most states, a pattern that has continued: in 1997, the average state paid 43 percent of the amount paid by private insurers for normal childbirth.[9] The result of this was low access to mainstream providers, precisely the situation Medicaid was meant to resolve. Many Medicaid patients therefore continued to utilize traditional forms of institutional care—clinics or safety-net or public hospitals rather than private doctors' offices.

And even though enrollment grew explosively, the states kept Medicaid a program for welfare recipients only, despite the hopes of its sponsors in 1965. Medicaid still did not enroll most poor children in most states in the 1960s, 1970s, and 1980s, and the legislative requirements that states move toward liberalized eligibility and comprehensive medical coverage for those who were enrolled were soon dropped.[10] Medicaid budgets were booming in the late 1960s and early 1970s, but this was in large part because of sharp increases in both the number of poor single-parent families and the proportion of those families who signed up for welfare, which went from 60 percent to 90 percent.[11]

The dominance of cost concerns in the Medicaid program was reflected in the slow implementation of the Early and Periodic

Screening, Diagnosis and Treatment program. EPSDT, passed in 1967, gave Medicaid children coverage for comprehensive well-child visits and preventive care. Both the Nixon administration, which failed to write regulations until 1971, and the states, which then took years to implement the program, sought to avoid the relatively modest costs involved. (A Democratic-majority Congress continued to push the program, but it took until 1976 for even a million children to get screenings out of more than 10 million who were eligible.[12]) The only optional Medicaid service in which all states enthusiastically participated immediately after it was passed in 1965—Medicaid assumption of Medicare Part B premiums for the low-income elderly—represented a net cost reduction for the states, shifting costs to the federal Medicare program that would otherwise be covered by Medicaid.[13]

Just as Medicaid enrollment had boomed with AFDC enrollment in the late 1960s and early 1970s, it stagnated with the welfare rolls in the late 1970s and early 1980s as states sought to cut costs in both programs and as the federal government lowered eligibility ceilings. Medicaid enrollment hit 22 million in 1975 and stayed at that level or below it for twelve years, until the federally mandated expansions of the late 1980s took effect, so that by 1987 only about 34 percent of the poor were covered by Medicaid.[14] At the same time, Medicare's enrollment continued to escalate steadily.

Post-Welfare Medicaid: 1988–2001

The first substantial expansions to Medicaid eligibility took place in the mid-1980s, with Congress mandating coverage of AFDC-eligible pregnant women and giving states a series of options to broaden eligibility to poor children, pregnant women, and seniors not on welfare. As with optional eligibility extensions in the original 1965 legislation, most states were slow to take advantage. A series of Medicaid expansions between 1984 and 1990 followed a repeated pattern: Congress authorized coverage options expansions for poor and near-poor women and children; most states failed to take advantage of them; Congress then made the coverage mandatory. Coverage of poor pregnant women and infants became mandatory in 1988, and uniform Medicaid eligibility was expanded to a variety of poor or near-poor women, children, and seniors in 1989 and 1990.

At that point, most states did become more aggressive in their eligibility rules for pregnant women and infants, with many increasing eligibility beyond the federally required income standard of 133 percent of poverty or lower. Thirteen states also exceeded mandates for some or all children aged one and up. These developments show significant legislative support for health insurance expansion in many states when the target population is compelling and when legislation gets a push from the federal government, a pattern that would recur in the past few years with the CHIP program for children in families with near-poor incomes. And these expansions, both voluntary and mandated, had a substantial impact: enrollment grew from 23 million in 1988 to 36 million in 1996.

But the Medicaid expansions also introduced a major new program failing: millions of pregnant women and children eligible for benefits but not enrolled. In 1996, only 58 percent of the children eligible for Medicaid under the expanded rules used it, while 77 percent of those children eligible for Medicaid under pre-expansion rules were enrolled. (The latter is a figure in line with other means-tested programs.)[15] This meant that 4.7 million uninsured children—40 percent of all uninsured children—were eligible for free health coverage but were not taking advantage of it.

Although governors and state legislators added some optional coverage to these Medicaid mandates, particularly for pregnant women and infants, state administrations disliked them overall. In the summer of 1989, forty-eight governors asked the federal government not to pass any more mandated expansions in Medicaid coverage. (The only governor who openly refused to sign was, typically, the governor of New York, Mario Cuomo.) Congress passed phased-in mandates for all poor children in 1990 anyway. Governor Bill Clinton of Arkansas complained that "the poorest states in country are going to have to pick up the biggest tab. . . . Nobody thought about what the practical impacts are." A senior Florida Medicaid administrator later recalled: "I remember our Medicaid program growing, and we thought, 'When does it end? . . . It was like Aliens IV. . . . Every time you thought you killed it, and it was slowing down, it knocked down the door, and you ran back, and Sigourney Weaver didn't have a shot.' It was terrible."[16]

State policymakers had reason to feel besieged. These expansions in child and maternity coverage occurred during what was already a period of rapid increases in Medicaid costs—142 percent between 1988 and 1993. Yet, although the new congressional mandates bore the brunt of criticism from the states, they were actually responsible for only 8.5 percent of that growth.[17] Young women and children are relatively inexpensive to cover, particularly compared to the elderly and disabled who incur the great majority of Medicaid's expenses. The real drivers of the boom in cost were broader health care cost inflation, growth in the numbers of elderly and disabled people on Medicaid, and the effects of the AIDS epidemic. Still, some states' officials saw their enrollment of pregnant women and children booming at the same time as their Medicaid costs and drew a mistaken connection. As we will see, reluctance in some states to enroll aggressively as their programs were growing was partly responsible for the failure of the Medicaid to reach almost half of those who gained eligibility.

The problem of underenrollment spread to Medicaid's original welfare base with the end of AFDC in 1997. With welfare reform causing millions of women to leave the welfare rolls that had previously provided an automatic link with Medicaid, many lost Medicaid coverage for themselves and their children despite their continued legal eligibility. Welfare-related Medicaid enrollment fell almost 40 percent from June 1997 to December 1999 in the twenty-one states with available data, 1.6 million in those states alone.[18] Even after controlling for the effects of the economic expansion, the number of children enrolled in Medicaid dropped between 926,000 and 1.37 million from 1995 to 1998, while the probability of a child with unemployed parents or in very poor families having Medicaid dropped significantly.[19] A recent study indicated that a large majority of women and children who lose Medicaid coverage after leaving welfare remain uninsured rather than receiving private health insurance.[20] As with other parameters pertaining to state health programs, these national statistics hide substantial variation: while Medicaid participation since welfare reform has suffered large declines among parents and children in New York and Texas, compounding already serious underenrollment problems, it has had impressive increases in several states, including traditionally conservative states like South Carolina and Indiana.[21]

In addition to underenrollment, both of the other issues that limited Medicaid's impact in the 1970s and 1980s—unambitious eligibility levels and underpayment of doctors—remain problematic today in many states. Many continue to be conservative with their levels of formal eligibility even though the federal government will pick up 50–70 percent of the cost. While federal mandates now require all states to cover poor children, as Figure 2.1 shows (see page 16), as of 2001 only fourteen states covered the parents of children in all poor families, with thirty-two setting income eligibility levels for parents at one minimum-wage salary or lower and several states excluding parents who make more than $4,000 a year, an amount that would not cover a typical family health insurance policy even if families devoted their entire income to premiums. (In many states these levels are an extension of old welfare eligibility levels, although Medicaid has been de-linked from welfare since 1996.)

Most state Medicaid programs still tend to pay doctors relatively poorly. While federal statutes historically kept payments to hospitals and nursing homes close to private and Medicare rates, by 1995 Medicaid was paying 40 percent of what private insurers pay for doctor's office visits and two-thirds of what Medicare pays.[22] Medicaid pays dentists even more poorly, covering only 10 percent of their costs.[23] There is a lot of state-to-state variation behind these numbers: when Medicaid fees are compared to local Medicare reimbursement for the same services, states vary from paying about 30 percent of Medicare fees in New York and New Jersey to more than 125 percent in Arkansas.[24] But, as Figure 2.2 shows (see page 17), the bottom line is that Medicaid does not pay doctors what Medicare and private insurers pay in the great majority of states.

Many doctors will not accept Medicaid, in large part as a result of the inadequacy of its payments (although some doctors may not want poor people in their offices). In a 1991 survey conducted by the American Medical Association, more than 60 percent of doctors said that they either will not see Medicaid patients or strictly limit how many they will see, and in a 1990 study 60 percent of pregnant Medicaid beneficiaries received prenatal care in clinics or other institutional settings, two and a half times the rate of other pregnant mothers.[25] Variation among states is substantial: while more than a third of physicians receive virtually no revenue from Medicaid in New Jersey—one of the lowest-paying Medicaid programs in the country—and the median New Jersey physician gets only 2 percent of income from the program, almost all physicians in Ohio (where payment averages 70 percent of what they get from Medicare) count at least a portion of their revenue from the program, and the median physician receives 10 percent.[26]

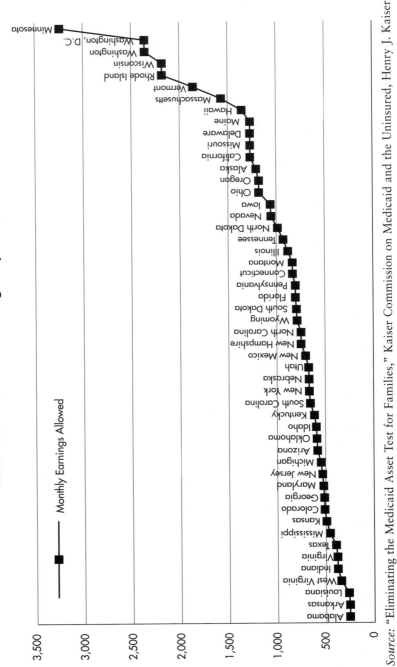

Figure 2.1
State Variation in Medicaid Eligibility for Parents

Source: "Eliminating the Medicaid Asset Test for Families," Kaiser Commission on Medicaid and the Uninsured, Henry J. Kaiser Family Foundation, Washington, D.C., April 2001.

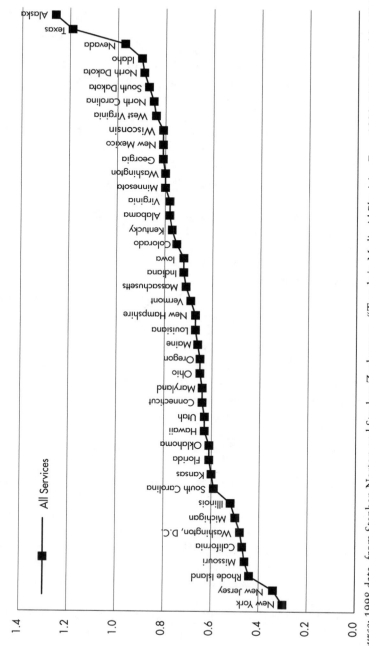

Figure 2.2

Medicaid vs. Medicare Payments to Doctors: Medicaid Is Almost Always Lower

Source: 1998 data, from Stephen Norton and Stephen Zuckerman, "Trends in Medicaid Physician Fees, 1993–1998," *Health Affairs* 19, no. 4 (July/August 2000): 222–32.

This phenomenon takes different forms in different places in the country. In many states, Medicaid, partly excluded from the mainstream of private physician offices, has instead become the best source of payment for "safety-net" providers—community health centers and clinics in public hospitals and urban academic hospitals. In most areas, Medicaid patients are either a burden on private physicians (a burden that many try to limit or exclude), the primary clientele for "Medicaid mill" physicians in high-poverty areas, or the cash cow for charity providers that otherwise treat the uninsured, illegal immigrants, and others whom no one else will see. Perhaps the worst performer on this score is New York, where Medicaid payment to doctors is the lowest in the country despite an otherwise very generous (and expensive) Medicaid program: a large number of Medicaid beneficiaries use emergency rooms for basic primary care, more than any other group in New York including the uninsured.[27]

The major effort to respond to this problem in the past ten to twelve years has been Medicaid managed care. In the late 1980s and early 1990s, almost all states began to shift a significant portion of their Medicaid beneficiaries into some sort of managed care plan. The percentage of Medicaid beneficiaries enrolled in managed care went from 10 percent in 1990 to 57 percent at the end of 2000. Most states have enrolled children and parents into private HMOs, paying them a flat per person monthly fee ("capitation") to cover Medicaid services. (A smaller number of states have employed less complete forms of privatization that leave the state as the insurer, while an even smaller number of states have privatized even more and enrolled most elderly and disabled Medicaid beneficiaries into HMOs.)

Medicaid managed care was intended to improve access to mainstream primary care in two ways: first, as the name "managed care" is meant to imply, these insurers would encourage patients' appropriate use of preventive and diagnostic services; second, Medicaid would enroll beneficiaries into mainstream insurance plans with large private sector enrollments, which would force their network of doctors to accept them as patients (the evocative technical term for this is "cram-down").

But Medicaid managed care also was intended to save money in almost all the states that pursued it.[28] Both private employers and state Medicaid programs were moving to HMOs because managed care promised to reduce or reverse the cost increases that had been hammering buyers of health care during the late 1980s and early 1990s. The problem is that the main way that managed care saves money is by reducing payment to doctors, hospitals, and other providers—negotiating lower rates in selective contracts with specific providers, reviewing expensive treatment decisions, shifting the financial risk for enrollee expenses onto doctors through capitation (paying a fixed per patient fee), and in some cases simply not paying some of their bills. That meant that Medicaid managed care was supposed to increase access to physicians at the same time that it saved money largely at their expense.

There is conflicting and incomplete evidence on whether Medicaid managed care has helped improve access to mainstream care.[29] That may be because Medicaid managed care has been variably effective at best at mainstreaming enrollees. While some states were willing to pay relatively high capitation rates to attract mainstream commercial plans (that is, plans not specializing in Medicaid coverage) as their programs got started and in the process were prepared to take a loss on Medicaid managed care, most states tried to pay less than their existing per enrollee costs to managed care plans, and those costs had already built in payment to doctors that was broadly considered inadequate. States varied hugely in the rates they would pay plans—from $82.75 per enrollee a month in California to $182.52 in Connecticut in 1998—and this variation bore little relation to local market conditions.[30] A 1999 study compared Medicaid managed care rates in thirty-five states (and the District of Columbia) to the rates Medicare managed care paid in the same states, a good proxy for health care costs in each state.[31] The study found almost no correlation between what Medicaid programs paid and what Medicare paid, as Medicaid payments to plans were based mostly on how well the program had previously paid providers and on whether states were putting a higher priority on saving money or on attracting commercial plans in their implementation of managed care. Although Medicaid managed care attracted strong participation from commercial plans through the early and mid-1990s, by the late 1990s, commercial plan participation in Medicaid managed care began dropping noticeably, so that 40 percent of Medicaid managed care enrollees were in Medicaid-dominated plans.[32] In many states, moreover, commercial plans providing Medicaid managed care use a separate network of providers for their Medicaid clients, in part because they could not or would not employ a "cram-down" of lower-paying Medicaid enrollees on their existing doctors and in part because their existing networks had few or no physician offices in low-income areas that have long been served exclusively by emergency rooms and Medicaid/charity care providers. Managed care, then, is no panacea for Medicaid's long-standing problems of under-reimbursement and lack of access to physicians.

1986–Present: QMB/SLMB

The QMB/SLMB, or "Medicare Buy-in" program seeks to reduce or eliminate out-of-pocket Medicare cost sharing for the low-income elderly. As with the other Medicaid expansions of the mid-1980s, the program began as a state option, in which states could use their Medicaid program to pay Medicare cost-sharing fees for seniors whose incomes were low but above Medicaid eligibility levels. And, as with the other 1980s Medicaid initiatives, voluntary state participation was minimal—only three states took part.

In 1988, the Medicare Buy-in program became mandatory for states.[33] The program was expanded to give more limited financial benefits to higher-income beneficiaries with the SLMB program in 1990 and the Qualified Individuals (QI) program in 1997.

These programs have been sharply limited by underenrollment problems. Because of ambiguous government data definitions in the QMB part of the program, it is hard to pin down even basic figures like total enrollment. Enrollment estimates in recent years have ranged from as low as 367,000 to as high as 2.4 million, while estimates of the eligible population ranged from 3 million to 5.1 million.[34] With both the numerator and the denominator uncertain, QMB participation rate estimates range from 15 percent to about 60 percent. Enrollment in SLMB benefits for seniors with incomes between 100 percent and 120 percent of the poverty line is clearly only between 200,000 and 300,000 enrollees, representing about 14–16 percent of those eligible. And the benefits allocated to seniors in the 1997 QI

---

* A program that allows Medicare beneficiaries to enroll in HMOs and pays the HMOs a rate based largely on Medicare's local costs. About 6 million Medicare beneficiaries are enrolled.

program (combining an extension of SLMB benefits to 135 percent of the poverty mark and a refund of some small Medicare fee increases for low-income seniors) demonstrate an extreme version of the underenrollment problem: at the end of 1998, the first year of the QI program, only 1 percent of the money set aside for it had been used and only 3 percent of potential participants had been enrolled.[35] While enrollment into the Medicare Buy-in program is weak in most states, there is a great deal of interstate variation: Mississippi and Massachusetts enroll more than 100 percent of the estimated number of low-income Medicare beneficiaries, while Rhode Island and Alaska enroll less than 5 percent, in one set of estimates.[36] Many states do not make even minimal efforts to keep track of potential "eligibles": as of 1999, only twenty states received data available monthly from HCFA that identifies low-income individuals newly enrolled in Medicare, and among those states that received the data, only twelve used it.[37]

1997–Present: CHIP

A bipartisan majority created the State Children's Health Insurance Program in 1997, sending money to states to cover children from families with incomes up to 200 percent of poverty or even higher and continuing the efforts to cover children that began in the mid-1980s. The program sought to provide more than $40 billion in federal matching funds over ten years.

By the beginning of 2001, all fifty states and the District of Columbia had begun enrolling children in CHIP programs. Medicaid and CHIP together should in principle cover up to three-quarters of the uninsured children in the United States and better than 90 percent of the low-income uninsured.[38] But despite the CHIP legislation and earlier Medicaid expansions, restrained health cost inflation, and the best economic climate in a generation, 2000 Census Bureau data showed that the number of children lacking coverage has remained high. (See Figure 2.3, page 22.) The number of uninsured children initially grew substantially after CHIP came into effect—from 9.8 million (13.8 percent) lacking coverage in 1995 to 11.1 million (15.4 percent) in 1998. In 1999 the figure for children without insurance fell almost back to its 1995 percentage, 13.9 percent, and in 2000 it fell further to 12.9 percent, lower than 1995 (though somewhat higher than it was in 1992), seemingly a

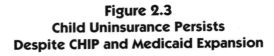

Figure 2.3
Child Uninsurance Persists
Despite CHIP and Medicaid Expansion

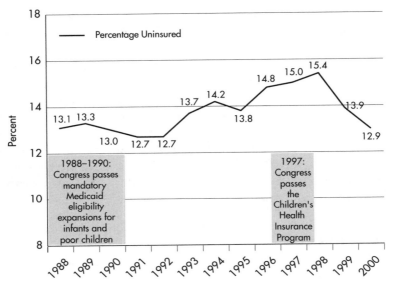

Source: Bureau of the Census, Current Population Survey, "Health Insurance Historical Tables," September 2001; available at www.census.gov/hhes/hlthins/historic/histt2.html.

major accomplishment. But this was a result of increased employer-based coverage; government health coverage remained at 23.2 percent of children, slightly lower than the percentage in 1997 just before CHIP began and substantially lower than the pre–welfare reform figure of 26.4 percent in 1995.[39] The 1999–2000 drop in the ranks of uninsured children is less than meets the eye: while CHIP gains no more than replaced reductions in child Medicaid enrollment, at its peak the booming economy reversed some of the erosion in employer coverage that had been experienced throughout the early and mid-1990s—an achievement that is likely already a pleasant memory. (See Figure 2.4, page 23.)

CHIP was a high-profile program when it was passed, but it then turned into something of a high-profile problem. Forty states did not use their full federal funding for 1998 by the end of fiscal year 2000 because of underenrollment problems, although states

Figure 2.4
Percentage of Children Covered by Health Insurance:
Public Coverage of Children Down, Private Coverage Up Since 1995

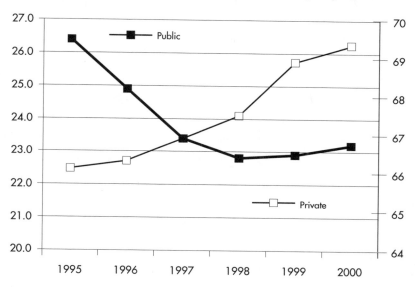

Source: Bureau of the Census, Current Population Survey, "Health Insurance Historical Tables," September 2001; available at www.census.gov/hhes/hlthins/historic/histt2.html. (2000 figures, unpublished, Bureau of Census analysis.)

were given three years to use the first year's allocation to give them time to get programs up and running. Those forty states were in principle required to forfeit those funds to the ten states that have spent their allotments, but Congress gave them a multiyear extension in late 2000. Some 1.5–2.3 million eligible children are not enrolled in CHIP, in addition to the 4.6–4.7 million children who are eligible for Medicaid but not yet enrolled.[40] The proportion of children eligible for either Medicaid or CHIP who actually enrolled was 42 percent in 1998–99.[41]

CHIP did grow rapidly in 2000. Total national enrollment jumped from 1.3 million to 2.7 million in the year and a half between June 1999 and December 2000.[42] Although CHIP is a small program, hundreds of thousands of uninsured children gained coverage in each of the states of California, New York, and Florida between the end of 1998 and December 2000, the date of the most recent enrollment figures. These are encouraging trends, and they are appearing in ever more places. While 35 percent of the growth in CHIP enrollment between June 1999 and June 2000, and 34 percent of total enrollment as of June 2000, was in three states that had substantial child health insurance programs before CHIP was passed (Florida, New York, and Pennsylvania), in late 2000 new initiatives in California and Texas drove the program's growth with hundreds of thousands of children covered.

As with Medicaid, there is substantial divergence in the operations and performance of CHIP programs. This belies simple geographic or ideological distinctions: Missouri has enrolled twice as many children into its CHIP program as has Michigan, although Missouri had less than half as many uninsured children from low-income families before the program started.[43] Similarly, although they are both conservative Southern states with similar populations and pre-CHIP levels of children lacking insurance, Georgia has enrolled three and a half times as many children into its CHIP program as has Virginia.[44]

Nevertheless, CHIP is broadly popular, more so than the much larger Medicaid program in many states. Virtually all states have used much simpler enrollment and reenrollment procedures for CHIP than they traditionally used for Medicaid, and they also have aggressively advertised the program. (In many states, CHIP rollout has been the occasion for simplifying Medicaid enrollment for children as well.)[45] Medicaid was long tied to welfare, and many states made joining the program difficult as an adjunct of their efforts to prevent welfare fraud and discourage welfare enrollment. A lot of states made Medicaid enrollment easier for nonwelfare pregnant women and children as the program expanded to reach those populations in the 1990s, and in most states there has been a pronounced shift in mentality toward increasing enrollment into CHIP, at least so far.[46] Additional pressure on states came because CHIP funding took the form of a block grant rather than an open-ended entitlement, so states with low enrollment risked forfeiting CHIP funding, as mentioned previously, a story that received a fair amount of attention in the local and national press.

Most states chose to use most or all CHIP funding for separate CHIP programs rather than expanding Medicaid, in part because of the stigma Medicaid has long had for potential enrollees, physicians, and for state politicians themselves.[47] Every one of these non-Medicaid CHIP programs dropped the Medicaid requirement of an in-person enrollment interview in a welfare office. Almost all the states dropped the requirement (applied in most Medicaid programs) that potential enrollees document their lack of assets, one of the greatest hassles in the Medicaid sign-up process in most states.

The mentality shift in favor of enrollment also shows up in new marketing and outreach spending. Medicaid programs had rarely advertised or otherwise sought to boost enrollment, though some states had begun to do so with the push to recruit pregnant women and infants for preventive care in the Medicaid expansions of the early 1990s. But many states did advertise their CHIP programs, and that inspired some of them to promote Medicaid for the first time as well.[48]

Most states, then, have been working strenuously to enroll children in CHIP. They have been doing so in what was until recently a uniquely favorable fiscal environment, as health inflation was quiescent in the late 1990s, Medicaid rolls dropped as a concomitant of welfare reform, and the economic boom and the tobacco settlement swelled their budgets. Still, there is an eligible, unenrolled child for almost every child that has been registered for CHIP. CHIP made significant gains in 2000 but only starting from a small base. CHIP and Medicaid expansion combined have barely been able to keep pace with the decline in employer coverage of children since 1988, never mind reduce the incidence of children going without insurance (or cut it in half, as backers of CHIP initially hoped).

State Drug Assistance Programs

As of May 2001, twenty-one states had programs to cover some or all prescription drug expenses for the poor elderly. (Missouri offers a small tax credit for seniors' drug expenses, and several other states force drug companies to sell at reduced prices to Medicare enrollees.) These programs are not on the Medicaid model because they are not federally mandated—they are the kind of voluntary state health insurance initiatives repeatedly folded into Medicaid model state-federal partnerships in the past forty years, and President Bush has proposed to do precisely that with state prescription drug programs. State drug assistance programs address a problem that Congress has repeatedly failed to deal with despite multiple opportunities. Yet, even though these programs are state-

sponsored initiatives, most manifest underenrollment and underfunding problems. They all have relatively generous income
ceilings—between $10,000 and $20,000 a year—that would in principle incorporate a substantial minority of seniors.[49] Yet all the state
programs put together covered about 2 percent of Medicare beneficiaries in 2000, and only three of the plans have enrollment of
more than 100,000, those of Pennsylvania, New Jersey, and New
York—they represent more than two-thirds of total national enrollment.[50] The rest of the programs are tiny. Yet the Bush administration proposes to build on this shaky foundation in its prescription
drug plan for the elderly. With prescription drugs, as elsewhere, the
poor performance of state-run, means-tested health coverage
schemes is no deterrent to policymakers in Washington. (Even the
three sizable programs may have underenrollment problems:
Pennsylvania's program is the largest, with about 200,000 beneficiaries in 2001. Yet this enrollment has been steadily dropping from
its high of close to 500,000 in the late 1980s.[51] New York State
projected enrollment of 475,000—out of 1.4 million eligible
seniors—when it created the Elderly Pharmaceutical Insurance
Coverage program in 1986.[52] By 1999, only 100,000 seniors were
signed up, although a recent large eligibility expansion has apparently increased enrollment to about 200,000 in 2001, still a fraction
of the now even greater pool of eligible seniors.)

As with CHIP, the underenrollment problem here cannot easily be explained by state disinterest. After all, states initiated these
programs, although the interest groups and politicians that were
behind such initiatives may not be the ones who can shape enrollment practices. Prescription drug coverage for seniors is politically
popular, particularly among the elderly, who vote in large numbers.

The lack of participation in CHIP and drug assistance efforts is
a sign that states may have trouble reaching middle- to low-income
people with health coverage programs even when state governments
fully buy into them politically. And the strong political commitment to CHIP is the exception in any event—most notably, we have
seen that many states cannot or will not spend the money neces-
sary to give Medicaid beneficiaries access to mainstream medical
care. As the next chapter shows, there are multiple, fundamental
reasons for these failures. They are pitfalls that states find difficult
to avoid even with concerted, good-faith efforts.

3

WHY THE MEDICAID MODEL FALLS SHORT, AND WHY WE KEEP EXPANDING IT ANYWAY

State-administered, means-tested health coverage suffers from consistent underenrollment, low levels of formal eligibility, and underpayment to physicians and private insurers. As the CHIP program's development thus far—enthusiastic efforts by many states leading to underwhelming enrollment numbers and little reduction in the ranks of the uninsured—makes especially clear, underenrollment does not necessarily result from state policy decisions, intentional or not. That is not true for under-reimbursement and low levels of formal eligibility. This chapter will explore some possible explanations for the persistent failures of these programs, beginning with an examination of the less political sources of underenrollment (problems 1 and 2) and then dealing with the politics of means-tested health coverage in the states and in Washington (problems 3–5).

WHY THE MEDICAID MODEL FALLS SHORT: FIVE UNDERLYING PROBLEMS

Means Testing Is a Formidable Enrollment Barrier

As we have seen, with all the attention to recruiting low-income families, almost 7 million eligible children were not enrolled in Medicaid and CHIP according to recent data The huge drop in the

27

welfare rolls in the late 1990s provides an important part of the explanation, as noted previously: welfare used to provide an automatic link with Medicaid, and now Medicaid and several similar programs are trying to reach people not on cash assistance. But that is a problem only likely to get worse as welfare time limits kick in for more and more beneficiaries. More broadly, most of the people who lack health coverage in America today are not part of the welfare system: they are children and adults in working families and senior citizens with some retirement income who cannot afford prescription drugs and Medicare cost sharing. Medicaid, CHIP, QMB/SLMB, and state prescription drug programs have had trouble reaching people who are unused to applying for programs geared to support the poor and are unwilling or unable to make a repeated effort to document their eligibility. Such programs are the wrong vehicle to reach the uninsured unless they are changed dramatically.

Problem 1: Working people and retirees are not aware of or comfortable with "welfare" health programs. Means-tested programs must enroll either low-income workers who are not expecting to be eligible for a government program and are not attentive to information about them or the nonworking poor, now frequently cut off from the cash welfare system that used to funnel them into Medicaid. Workers and retirees also are often reluctant to participate in means-tested "welfare" programs and skeptical of the quality of care they will receive on "welfare insurance."[1] And even disregarding their welfare association, small, targeted programs must overcome a basic name-recognition problem. For these reasons, many working people are not aware that they or their children are eligible for public coverage: one study found that six out of ten parents whose children qualify for CHIP or Medicaid do not believe the program applies to them and that 82 percent of these parents said they would enroll their children if they knew they qualified.[2]

Problem 2: Means testing makes it hard to enroll people because of paperwork to verify eligibility initially and at repeated intervals. The cumbersome process associated with income and asset verification also serves to limit enrollment. Almost 40 percent of families with eligible but uninsured children had tried to apply for Medicaid at least once and either had been denied coverage or had failed to complete the application.[3] Medicaid and QMB/SLMB applications in some states are dozens of pages long, although they were shortened for nonwelfare children in many states after Medicaid was separated from welfare. This poses a barrier even for those who make it through the paperwork—the General Accounting Office found that half of all denied Medicaid applications in the early 1990s were the result of a failure to provide required documentation rather than actual ineligibility.[4] Moreover, states require enrollees to re-verify their eligibility regularly to continue in the programs, resulting in a great deal of churning as individuals move on and off the rolls. This happens because individuals' incomes fluctuate, because they fail to fill out what can be long applications to renew coverage, or because each "recertification" is another opportunity for bureaucracies to make a processing mistake.

In some cases these enrollment barriers can be totally impenetrable. A survey of Medicare beneficiaries in New York City who qualified for the QMB/SLMB program but were not enrolled found that almost 90 percent of them had never heard of it.[5] This is hardly surprising—New York, like most states, makes no effort to publicize the program besides placing fliers in government offices.[6] But the more remarkable result came in a follow-up effort that tracked participants to see if they enrolled in the program once they had learned about it: fewer than 10 percent received the benefit after a year.[7] Many did not apply, in part because the application process involves extensive asset documentation and two separate face-to-face meetings at a Medicaid office. And those who did apply found that most Medicaid office staff were unable or unwilling to give out program information on QMB/SLMB, even when professional advocates accompanied them to the office.

Nevertheless, most states have backed off the most egregious enrollment and reenrollment hassles, particularly in bringing children into Medicaid and CHIP. (These barriers were generally a holdover from Medicaid's welfare connection.) While many states used to require recertification every six months, and some every three, now thirty-nine states review eligibility every twelve months for children.[8] Forty states no longer require applicants for children's coverage to come to a welfare or Medicaid office for a face-to-face interview, either at initial enrollment or at reenrollment, and forty-two states have stopped requiring applicants for child coverage to have no or minimal assets to be eligible. Several more states have dropped these requirements for CHIP applicants but not for Medicaid applicants, making such simplifications nearly universal in the CHIP program.

Yet, despite these efforts, underenrollment persists. Some have used the evidence of shortfalls in state health program performance as grounds for criticizing state responsibility as such for Medicaid and similar programs.[9] At least when it comes to underenrollment, though, means testing itself, rather than state administration, is a major part of the problem. Means testing does not preclude enrollment of most or all potential beneficiaries, but it does make it difficult. Governments—state or federal—will only achieve widespread participation if they make that goal a sustained, high priority. In most states, means-tested health program enrollment has not been that kind of priority except for brief periods, for the political reasons to be discussed later in this chapter. So underenrollment results from a combination of the practical difficulties and programmatic requirements of income verification and the lack of political will in most states to ease those requirements enough to gather in everyone eligible.

Medicare enrolled virtually its entire target population in its first year of operation, as noted earlier. It avoided means testing and its attendant problems. The Social Security system allowed almost automatic Medicare enrollment, with only a nominal step required for Part B participation. Medicare, moreover, is conceptualized as an earned social insurance benefit—it has no "welfare stigma," and it is politically one of the strongest programs in American history. If states made Medicaid enrollment truly easy, they would risk allowing people with excessively high incomes onto the rolls and displacing private coverage, a politically objectionable outcome for a program conceptualized as a welfare benefit. Underenrollment has often (although not always) been a problem for means-tested programs funded and operated by the federal government, even programs with broad political support such as Head Start.* (States control enrollment into Medicaid and related programs with loose guidelines and supervision from Washington.)

---

*One important exception is Supplementary Security Income, a national program that provides a minimum income to the blind, disabled, and elderly who can show eligibility (including income eligibility). When the Nixon administration initiated the program in the early 1970s, it was administered directly by the federal Social Security Administration, and overenrollment resulted: SSA was overwhelmed with eligibility determination, and responsibility was shifted to the states with SSA oversight under federal eligibility rules. (See Peter Passell and Leonard Ross, *State Policies and Federal Programs: Priorities and Constraints* [New York: Twentieth

But if the difficulties of means testing were totally overwhelming the good intentions of the states to enroll the eligible, operational differences between the states' programs would not matter much. Yet there is striking evidence that states can do a better job on enrollment. Vermont, a state with relatively low per capita income, has achieved universal coverage for children and 90 percent coverage for its whole population with means-tested public health insurance and strenuous marketing efforts. Vermont has a lower level of private coverage than nearby Maine, but half Maine's proportion of uninsured residents is in its low-income population thanks to its public program enrollment.[10] As will be shown in more detail below, the main difference in Vermont seems to be the political will to do what it takes to approach universal coverage, starting with the current governor, Howard Dean, a physician who is strongly committed to public health. The difference operational decisions can make is particularly clear when it comes to specific programs: Missouri, South Carolina, New York, and Florida bucked the national trend and had excellent CHIP enrollments relative to need; Massachusetts and Mississippi drove up QMB/SLMB enrollment with aggressive outreach, while in most other states it languished.[11] Means testing may well make enrollment significantly harder than it is in a universal program like Medicare. But the way in which programs are implemented at the state level clearly does make a difference.

The problem of large populations who are "eligible but not enrolled," then, is also partly an issue of lack of policy innovation and lack of political will in the states. States can attract potential enrollees, but they have to do the tough job of overcoming the taint of association with welfare and the hassle of income verification. Most states have not made the political commitment to do so. Indeed, we will see that some states have explicitly committed themselves to holding down enrollments in their health programs. And

---

Century Fund, 1978], pp. 131–32.) And SSI has apparently not had underenrollment problems under state administration either, with between 80 percent and 90 percent of eligible people with work disabilities participating. (See Mitchell LaPlante et al., "Income and Program Participation of People with Work Disabilities," *Disability Statistics Report* no. 9, National Institute on Disability and Rehabilitation Research, U.S. Department of Education, April 1997.) Together with historically high enrollment levels for AFDC, this suggests that cash assistance programs may have an easier time enrolling people than means-tested service delivery programs for people with low or no incomes.

recall that the problems of stringent formal eligibility levels and inadequate reimbursement are exclusively the results of conscious political decisions in the states. The distinctive political and fiscal pressures on state government are therefore a critical piece of the explanation for shortfalls in the Medicaid model.

Underperformance and the Complex, Troubled Politics of Health Coverage in the States

Consider the following news item from Boise's *Idaho Statesman* on March 29, 2001:

SENATE LIMITS KIDS' HEALTH FUNDING; GOP VOTES TO CAP INSURANCE PROGRAM, LIMIT RECRUITMENT
By Bob Fick
The Associated Press

Senate Republicans overwhelmingly voted on Wednesday to slap a cap on subsidized health care for children of the working poor and ordered the Health and Welfare Department to drastically curtail efforts to let those families know they are eligible for the help.

The provision, part of the $800 million Medicaid budget, now goes to the House.

Sen. Robert Lee, who has been on a yearlong crusade to find some way of checking the growth of the Medicaid budget, argued that the department's aggressive campaign to identify children eligible for the Children's Health Insurance Program has turned up four times as many who qualify for Medicaid.

After starting off extremely slowly with just a few hundred children in 1997, participation in the past two years has skyrocketed to more than 10,000 children, whose families are too poor to afford health insurance but not poor enough to qualify for Medicaid. At the same time, the promotional effort has been credited with uncovering tens of thousands of new Medicaid participants.

By capping the participants in the children's health care program and then doing as little as possible to let people know the program exists, the Rexburg Republican said the state can rein in the explosive expansion of Medicaid rolls. Medicaid is costing taxpayers $204 million in state general tax revenue and another $516 million in federal money this year.

"We must face fiscal reality," Lee said, mirroring comments he made earlier in convincing legislative budget writers to endorse the approach. "It has the potential of really bankrupting the state."

Rep. Hod Pomeroy of Boise was the only one of the 18 Republicans on the Joint Finance-Appropriations Committee to join the two Democrats against limiting the reach of the Children's Health Insurance Program. Senate Democrats got little more support in that chamber.

"I can't understand why it is such an undesirable thing to let people know something is available," Democratic Sen. Lin Whitworth of Inkom said. "I cannot understand why you would provide a program for people sorely in need and hide it under a bushel."

Democratic Rep. Ken Robison of Boise maintained that spending the money on health care now would likely generate savings in taxpayer-borne medical expenses for the same people once they become sick.

"We ought to be interested in covering more children, not less," he said.

But the Senate agreed with the budget panel and denied the department the authority to tap into a $58 million surplus to cover children beyond those the current $21 million budget allows.

Although that money must either be spent on the health program or be returned to the federal government, lawmakers refused to use it because once it runs out the state would again be on the hook for either more state money or limiting participation then. They opted to impose the limits now, even if it means throwing some children off the program if participation exceeds the $21 million budget.

The Senate bill also prohibits the department from spending any other money to promote the insurance program. It is spending $658,000 from its welfare block grant to advertise the program.

Analysts say the state would meet the federal promotional requirement by simply issuing a brochure.

State legislators in Idaho are trying to prevent uninsured children from finding out they are eligible for Medicaid and CHIP—indeed, they could not be more explicit about it. For those who follow state health politics closely, this might be disappointing but not surprising. Yet the same circumstances would never happen in Medicare—fiscal hawks in Congress deciding to shut down publicity about the program in the hopes of leaving senior citizens uninsured. In fact, for anyone who follows American politics, it is nearly inconceivable. To make matters worse, the debate described above was actually about whether or not Idaho would use federal money to buy health insurance for children in low-income families (and risk spending more state money down the line) or would forfeit the federal money, leave the poor children uninsured, and cap its own potential spending.

Idaho is a conservative state. Al Gore received only 28 percent of the vote there in 2000, one of the four lowest totals in the nation for him. But even conservative Republicans in Congress—even Idaho Republicans—would never openly advocate cutting off enrollment of the elderly into Medicare the way they did children into Medicaid and CHIP. While the interests of the elderly are arguably more politically influential than the interests of children in both Washington, D.C., and Idaho, the shutdown of CHIP outreach in Idaho did not happen strictly because of the state's conservatism or because children lack the pull that seniors have. The federal legislation that created the State Children's Health Insurance Program was sponsored by Orrin Hatch, Republican senator of Utah. Al

Gore got just 26 percent of the vote in Utah, even less than in Idaho. Moreover, Idaho is only one of several states that openly sought to hold down Medicaid and CHIP enrollment in 2000 and 2001: North Carolina actually froze CHIP enrollment and started a waiting list; Kentucky reinstated and California kept in place income verification requirements, with California's Democratic governor tellingly describing his veto of a bill to remove those requirements as a spending issue rather than a fraud issue; Washington State, like Idaho, cut back on CHIP outreach efforts and nearly froze CHIP enrollment.[12] All this was after a period of unusually slow growth in Medicaid costs and strength in state budgets.

State health politics is different from national health politics, and Medicaid politics is different from Medicare politics as well. Medicaid and its policy cousins are administered by the states, while Medicare is administered federally. But there are other important differences: Medicaid, CHIP, and other, similar health programs are targeted at the poor or near-poor and paid for by both states and the federal government, while Medicare provides universal health coverage for the elderly and is paid for exclusively by the federal government. These differences have important consequences.

Problem 3: Programs without benefits to the middle class are politically weak in interest group politics. Fiscal conservatives in Washington are sometimes exasperated by the growth of Medicare expenditures, and they are not necessarily bashful about moving aggressively to get those costs under control. Indeed, it is one of the ironies in American health policy that it was the Reagan administration that adopted a big-government, centralized, administrative price-setting system for Medicare in the early 1980s as a way to cut spending growth, a system that now plays an enormous role in determining hospital and other health care prices in the United States. But federal policymakers must be very careful about any action that threatens cuts to beneficiaries or otherwise appears to impinge directly on their interests. Medicare beneficiaries have several well-organized and powerful voices in Washington, and Medicare is a tremendous issue in congressional and presidential elections.

In contrast, although elderly and disabled beneficiaries have some power as interest groups, the poor and near-poor who make up most state health program enrollees are seldom well organized or influential in the policy development process. Institutional providers like hospitals and nursing homes have the greatest lobbying power over these programs, and they also enjoyed a statutory federal guarantee of competitive reimbursement from Medicaid until recently. Since physicians and other outpatient providers usually get little revenue from Medicaid, they have neither tried nor had much success at raising Medicaid rates in most states to private or Medicare levels.

Problem 4: Health programs are marginal in state electoral politics. There is significant evidence that governors and legislators get little scrutiny in state elections for health care policy in general and even less for enrolling and covering low-income people. While health care routinely appears among the top two or three issues in exit polling in national elections, it almost never does in state elections. Exit polls often ask voters to rank their "top issues" in deciding their vote. In the 2000 national election, Medicare and health care received 15 percent of responses under "which issues matter most" (the most demanding question phrasing), tied for second with education.[13] In previous national elections, either health care or Medicare ranked as one of the top three issues in 1992–96 and as a major issue in 1998: health care was third in 1992 and 1994 and sixth in 1998, while Medicare was second in 1996. In contrast, in ten available exit polls in state elections in 1997–98 (the most recent cycle since state elections do not typically receive separate polling on issue priorities in presidential years like 2000), health care was not among the top issues in nine. The exception came when it placed fifth in California in 1998, and that for a category called "Health care/HMOs"—that is, an issue of regulation of private insurance rather than public insurance programs.[14]

State elections are instead dominated by the issues of education, crime, and, most important, taxes; exit polls show it, as do campaigning themes. The centrality of the tax issue helps to explain a striking disparity in national versus state elections in the country as a whole and particularly in the northeastern states. Republicans achieved a thorough dominance of the nation's governorships in the 1990s. Even New York, Massachusetts, Rhode Island, and Connecticut have Republican governors, although these states have become a virtual regional lock for Democrats in national elections. In each one of these states, Republicans have won office promising tax cuts as their central agenda item.

There is a close relationship between problem 3—the political weakness of programs for low-income people—and problem 4, the irrelevance of health care policy in state public opinion and in state elections. Republicans at the state level can run on tax cuts without raising the specter of curtailing middle-class entitlements: this is particularly true in health care, in which federal programs are universal and state programs are targeted at the poor and near-poor. (Democrats have only recently rediscovered the middle-class issue of public education as a response to the dominance of taxes in state politics.) It is especially telling that the only health care issue to get on the radar screen of state politics in the second half of the 1990s was regulation of the HMOs that cover the insured middle class.

Problem 5: Poorer states face intense fiscal pressure, yet they have the greatest need. The centrality of tax cuts in state politics puts a great deal of fiscal pressure on state governments, and that pressure is intensified by constitutional requirements to balance the budget in most states. The rapid inflation in Medicaid costs in the early 1990s, driven largely by broader health care and long-term care cost inflation, further increased the fiscal squeeze on states. Twenty-five states enacted large tax increases to maintain balanced budgets between 1990 and 1992, in part because of Medicaid costs. Medicaid went from claiming 8.3 percent to 11.6 percent of state tax revenue between 1988 and 1992.[15] (Medicaid aficionados will want to verify that this excludes the state accounting gimmick using the Disproportionate Share Hospital Program to inflate Medicaid spending by setting reimbursement rates that take into account hospitals that serve a disproportionate number of the indigent whose needs are expensive to treat in order to run up federal matching dollars—it does.) The fiscal pressure on states takes a particularly heavy toll on health programs in relatively poor states. These states have the greatest potential demand on their Medicaid programs and other programs for the poor, and high crime rates and large numbers of children also create major demands on their budgets. They have the most money at risk if they adopt inclusive eligibility standards and enrollment practices for health programs and the least fiscal capacity to risk it.

Most poor states, particularly in the South, have broadly limited Medicaid programs: they pay low rates of reimbursement to providers for health care, do not cover many common Medicaid services, and enroll only a small percentage of their poor, uninsured population into the program. Nine of the twelve states in the Southeast have both below-average eligibility levels (relative to their poor population) and below-average spending per Medicaid enrollee, and Oklahoma, Alabama, Mississippi, and Texas had among the nation's most limited Medicaid programs in two recent surveys with different methodologies.[16] These states spend about one-third the national average in terms of Medicaid dollars per poor resident.

There is more than a conservative regional orientation behind these figures. Indeed, when rankings of state Medicaid program spending are adjusted for the demographic and fiscal resources of the states, the picture changes considerably. One report recently adjusted raw Medicaid spending figures in several ways: first, by comparing Medicaid spending to the number of low-income, non-privately insured state residents, the report generated a figure for spending per "individual at risk" for lacking insurance; then, the report compared such spending to state per capita income and to state taxation levels.[17] The new rankings show clearly that wealthy states with few low-income uninsured people (and therefore limited budget exposure) spend the most on them, and poor states with many low-income uninsured people spend the least per such person. Medicaid spending relative to need in roughly thirty-six out of fifty-one jurisdictions (including the District of Columbia) falls into a narrow band, varying mostly with per capita income (see Figure 3.1). Only three southeastern states fall below the band—Texas, Florida, and Virginia—while Tennessee and Kentucky are above it and North Carolina almost is.

A closer look at the states that vary from this band is telling, and the results confirm the political difficulty of raising taxes in states. States that spend a relatively large share of gross state product per capita on Medicaid mostly do it by shifting resources from other programs rather than by raising taxes. Looking at Medicaid spending relative to state income per head, while all of the top nineteen states are above average in the share of the budget they devote to Medicaid, they are all over the place in their tax rates.[18] With a few exceptions (Alaska, Hawaii, New Mexico, Delaware, West Virginia) these states have been willing to set up generous Medicaid programs, given their resources and the potential expense of providing for uninsured poor people, but they have not been willing to let taxes go up relative to other states to pay for it. And most of

Figure 3.1
States' Per Captia Income and Their Medicaid Spending Per Capita at Risk, 1999

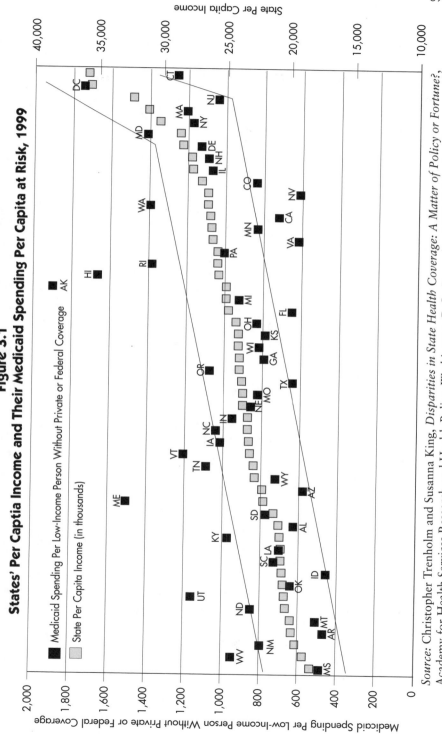
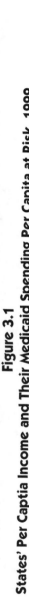

■ Medicaid Spending Per Low-Income Person Without Private or Federal Coverage

□ State Per Capita Income (in thousands)

Source: Christopher Trenholm and Susanna King, *Disparities in State Health Coverage: A Matter of Policy or Fortune?,* Academy for Health Services Research and Health Policy, Washington, D.C., December 2000, Tables 3 and 4 and Figure 1.

these states—in which Medicaid takes up an unusually big chunk of the budget—are relatively rich, meaning that they take some of the fiscal flexibility their wealth affords them and devote it to an extra-generous Medicaid program, leaving other programs at the level more typical of average states. The reverse is largely true of those states with low percentages of their budget devoted to Medicaid: they are mostly poor states that choose to squeeze Medicaid in order to maintain other programs at a level they could not afford otherwise, not states cutting Medicaid spending to maintain relatively low tax rates.

The progressive states. This largely deterministic picture seems to leave out an important group of states that approved broad, means-tested health expansions in the mid-1990s. These states—Tennessee, Oregon, Wisconsin, Minnesota, Washington, Vermont, Massachusetts, Rhode Island, and Delaware—have either pioneered efforts to give means-tested health insurance to nondisabled, working-age adults, a population almost entirely ignored in Washington, D.C., since 1994, or have dramatically extended coverage to parents (see Table 3.1). And the list includes wealthy states (Massachusetts, Minnesota, Washington, Rhode Island, and Delaware), average states (Wisconsin and Oregon), and low-income, low-tax states (Tennessee and Vermont). Do these states show that a national program modeled on their initiatives could bring us close to universal coverage?

What has happened in these states appears promising. Between 1994 and 1996 they extended health coverage to low- and middle-income parents and to childless adults with incomes up to 100–175 percent of the poverty line through Medicaid eligibility expansions and separate state-funded programs.

A closer look at these initiatives, however, shows that they are mostly relatively small programs in states with high levels of private coverage. (Levels of private coverage vary widely from state to state.) They are mostly variants of the dynamic described above: rich (and/or high private coverage) state—limited budget risk—expansive eligibility. In six of the nine states, Medicaid expansion has still left the state's Medicaid coverage of its nonelderly population about equal to or less than the national average.

Several of these states initially passed more ambitious plans for universal coverage, typically through an employer mandate. They all backed off those reforms, and in Washington, Oregon, Rhode

Table 3.1

STATE PERCENTAGE OF NONELDERLY POPULATION ON MEDICAID, 1997–99

STATE	PERCENTAGE
Wisconsin	5.7
Minnesota	7.7
Oregon	8.9
Delaware	9.0
Rhode Island	9.1
Washington	9.1
Massachusetts	11.5
Vermont	12.8
Tennessee	16.3
U.S	8.5

Source: "State Profiles 2001," AARP Public Policy Institute, Washington, D.C., 2002.

Island, and Tennessee, fiscal pressures have led governments to scale back partially the more limited means-tested expansions initiated in the mid-1990s.[19] Notably, most of these states never made an explicit political commitment to shift substantial state public resources and tax revenues into an attempt to provide universal coverage. The early 1990s health reform debate in most of them focused more on the need for centralized control of health cost inflation than on the need for universal coverage.[20] Finally, none of these expansions relied on general tax revenues. Instead, they were funded with health care provider taxes or "sin" taxes, mainly on cigarettes. Another round of modest state coverage enhancements arrived in the late 1990s with the windfall of the tobacco settlement. It is doubtful whether these kinds of special taxes and onetime revenue bursts could sustain programs with larger enrollments.

By far the largest and most consequential of these programs, with almost as many enrollees as the others put together, is

Tennessee's TennCare program.[21] TennCare, developed and implemented at the same time that the Clinton health care reform proposal went through its rise and fall in Washington, tremendously expanded enrollment into Medicaid in Tennessee to cover potentially all uninsured residents and all people with chronic conditions closed out of the insurance market while shifting enrollees into managed care. Consider, in contrast to the earlier news story from Idaho, the breathtaking developments in Tennessee criticized in this *Wall Street Journal* editorial:

Tennessee Reels
Wall Street Journal, June 21, 2000

. . . Last year, Governor Sundquist's tax proposal failed after horn-honking protestors in cars circled the Capitol building and three-fourths of Republicans in the state house opposed their own party's governor on the issue. But Mr. Sundquist is now back with his proposal to create a 3.75% income tax while reducing the state sales tax, and he vows to veto anything that isn't a "long-term solution to the tax structure."

Few people argue that Tennessee doesn't need tax and budget reforms. But many wonder why budget reform doesn't come first so Tennessee can continue to attract jobs as one of nine states without an income tax. State revenues are growing by 7% this year, yet the budget remains in deficit because the state's managed-care alternative to Medicaid now covers an amazing one out of four state residents and consumes 42% of the budget. But rather than tackle the radical overhaul of TennCare, Governor Sundquist and key Democratic legislators think an income tax is the answer to the budget's structural problems. . . . Tommy Hopper, a former political director of the Republican National Committee under Jim Nicholson, now heads the state's Free Enterprise Coalition. He says Governor Sundquist's proposed tax is suicide for the Republican Party. "I designed and wrote Sundquist's 1994 mailing that featured his opposition to an income tax," he says. "He of all people should know what a political weapon it can be against candidates."

TennCare is a genuine achievement. It has been maintained at substantial expense by a Republican governor and legislature, and it has covered enough uninsured Tennesseeans, despite low levels of private insurance coverage, to reduce the proportion of the population without insurance to 13.4 percent, a level far below that of states with similar levels of private coverage including Texas, New York, California, and neighboring Arkansas.[22] This state commitment has put the Republican governor, Don Sundquist, in the uncomfortable position of violating the most fundamental and ubiquitous party principle of at least the past fifteen years—opposition to income tax increases—and earning the angry disapproval of the *Wall Street Journal* in the process. (As of this writing, Sundquist is still fighting with the legislature over the issue.) And this is primarily in defense of a program that covers a quarter of all state residents, including hundreds of thousands of low-income, uninsured adults who have been neglected in Washington health policy legislation for decades.

But TennCare is an exception among these programs as a major fiscal and enrollment commitment. It is telling how little other state coverage expansions have necessitated the basic conversation about the size of government that has been raised by an undertaking on TennCare's scale. TennCare is a huge program—it caused Tennessee's Medicaid program to grow by more than 500,000 enrollees. But it has had serious problems retaining doctors and managed care plans, mainly because of low payment rates.[23] This culminated with the financial collapse of two large plans and the withdrawal, oft-threatened in the past, of Blue Cross/Blue Shield, by far the largest participating plan in terms of enrollment and its mainstream provider network. Budgetary pressure also has led TennCare to limit most new enrollment since 1995. Finally, and most discouraging, Governor Sundquist recently endorsed a restructuring of the program that would drop 180,000 enrollees and would reduce benefits for the remaining enrollees who are not part of the traditional Medicaid population. TennCare, then, is an important achievement, but it also is a fiscally troubled program, one that has established a difficult to maintain high-water mark for partial coverage rather than a down payment on universal coverage.

The most unambiguously promising of these programs are those in Massachusetts and Vermont. Their expansions have brought them close to universal coverage. The proportion of residents without insurance in Massachusetts is down to 5.9 percent, and lack of insurance among low-income Vermonters is at 15 percent, by far the lowest in the United States.[24] These states have defied the national patterns. Massachusetts, a rich state with a high incidence of private coverage, has taken on a major budgetary commitment in giving Medicaid to a significantly higher proportion of its residents than the national average, while Vermont, a much less prosperous state, has covered more of its low-income population than any other. But these are not typical states. They have unusual political orientations and congenial demographic circumstances. Their examples simply show that, in a liberal, wealthy state with very high private coverage levels (note that Massachusetts is well within the spending/income band in Figure 3.1) and in an even more liberal state with the second-smallest population in the country, it is possible to approach universal coverage using the Medicaid model. They are the exceptions that prove the more discouraging rule.

WHY WASHINGTON LOVES THE MEDICAID MODEL

So why are decentralized and highly targeted health insurance programs so politically appealing despite their apparently chronic limitations?

States Are Not "Big Government"

The first part of the answer is the curious tendency to differentiate between states and government. Even a casual observer of American politics knows that decisions about situating administrative power in the states or in Washington carry a great deal of ideological weight. Liberals have traditionally (and particularly since the civil rights era) distrusted states as politically regressive, and there is a liberal academic literature arguing that it is the result of a conscious effort by reactionary forces that American poverty programs, and particularly programs with the potential to help blacks economically, have been administered in the states since the 1930s.[25] The continuing popularity of state-administered health coverage expansions, though, can hardly be understood as race-driven, both because health insurance does not have the same social implications as income support did in the Jim Crow South and because in any event programs like CHIP and Medicaid expansion are explicitly directed at delinking public health coverage from income support. Nevertheless, there is a more fundamental ideological theme in American politics that gives a powerful impetus to this decentralizing tendency: the notion that states are governments closer to the people.

Americans are notoriously uncomfortable with government action in society and with the political conflict that follows on giving government the power to act explicitly and directly. That means that expressions of government power cannot be presented as such, at least not straightforwardly. The most high-profile recent manifestation of this phenomenon in health care policy was the Clinton administration's early choice for "managed competition" as a mechanism for national health insurance, ostensibly leaving government to set the rules for private insurers and semiprivate groups of consumers rather than provide or pay for care directly—an approach that nonetheless failed to assuage fears of a government takeover of health care. If the Medicare program seems like an exception, it is made possible in part because outsiders do not know the extent to which Medicare's payment rates and other policies are the subject of normal political conflict and negotiation.[26] It also became law in 1965, when Democrats had the presidency and an enormous majority in both houses of Congress.

The connection between American resistance to political conflict and direct government action on the one hand and devolution to states on the other has to do with the way Americans and the American media think about state governments as opposed to federal government. In 1996 and 1997, several prominent Republicans supported the State Children's Health Insurance Program but insisted on allowing states even more discretion than they have in Medicaid. Senator Orrin Hatch, principal Republican sponsor of the CHIP legislation, objected to a proposed Medicaid expansion as "nothing but a big bureaucracy and a big entitlement program" and insisted on loosening restrictions on states and turning the program from an entitlement (in which states would have to enroll anyone eligible) into a block grant (in which states could limit enrollment and control other basic parameters).[27] His reasoning was representative: the most common epithet tied to centralized, national administration of health programs is "big," and particularly "big government."

It is easy to poke holes in this logic—although Senator Phil Gramm of Texas during the CHIP debate rejected a "bureaucratic, Washington approach" and then "rejoice[d] that we might have 50 different plans," it is not particularly likely that fifty state programs would result in less bureaucracy than one national one.[28] But small governing units seem clearly to be a legitimizer in and of themselves in America: the smaller the scope of a government jurisdiction, the less intimidating and foreign it seems as an institution. Indeed, in debates over devolving health policy, those emphasizing the closeness of states to the people and the evils of Washington often seem to regard state government as not really government at all.

One recent exception to this romanticizing of state governments in Washington has been the cool reception Congress gave to President Bush's initial proposal on prescription drug coverage for seniors. Bush proposed a program of grants to states to offer means-tested coverage as an "immediate helping hand" in lieu of a broader Medicare prescription drug benefit—that is, he envisioned furnishing prescription drugs to seniors on the Medicaid model. Both congressional parties have been hostile. Charles Grassley, the Republican chairman of the Senate Finance Committee, refused even to consider the proposal, showing support instead for a federally run universal entitlement through Medicare. At the January 18, 2001, nomination hearing for Tommy Thompson as secretary of health and human services, Grassley weighed in with comments that have been echoed repeatedly by others in both parties in Congress:

> The President-elect's proposal you have heard talked about euphemistically here, that is, not in very glowing terms. That is, the Helping Hand block grant to States. I very much hope that you would take back to the President-elect the word that it is not going to be very favorably received here in Congress, and that we have an opportunity to really do more to help the American people. A lot of States really do not want to take on this additional responsibility. They have new programs thrust on them, similar to the one outlined by the President-elect. I think most of us want some form of universal coverage. I mean, after all, Medicare is universal. Why should prescription drug benefits not also be universal? . . . It just seems to me that if we have a proposal

for a universal tax cut, we certainly in America, at this point, with our large budget surpluses, could have a universal drug coverage benefit.

These are generic concerns, reflecting broad skepticism about the willingness of "a lot of states" to participate in new health programs and the wisdom of means-testing health benefits. They reflect an appreciation of the dangers of continual federal enlargement of state administrative responsibilities for health programs. The contrast between the enthusiasm for diluting federal control during legislative debate on CHIP and the reluctance to shift administration to the states when it comes to Medicare prescription drugs no doubt reflects the differences between the politics of Medicare—a program with a highly organized constituency that votes—and the politics of the nonelderly uninsured—who are poorly organized and vote in small numbers. But it also reflects at least some awareness in Washington that Medicaid expansion, CHIP, and similar initiatives have had real problems, problems that need to be addressed before we continue to channel expansions of public coverage into that model.

Means Testing Does Not Threaten the Privately Insured

In the immediate aftermath of the 1994 Republican landslide, preceded by the failure of his national health insurance plan, Bill Clinton made the following pronouncement in his 1995 State of the Union speech:

> I still believe our country has got to move toward providing health security for every American family. But I know that last year, as the evidence indicates, we bit off more than we could chew. So I'm asking you that we work together. Let's do it step by step. Let's do whatever we have to do to get something done. Let's at least pass meaningful insurance reform so that no American risks losing coverage for facing skyrocketing prices. That nobody loses their coverage because they face high prices or unavailable insurance, when they change jobs and lose a job, or a family member gets sick. . . . We ought to make sure that self-employed people in small businesses can buy insurance at more affordable rates through voluntary purchasing pools. We ought to help

families provide long-term care for a sick parent or a disabled child. We can work to help workers who lose their
jobs at least keep their health insurance coverage for a year
while they look for work. And we can find a way—it may
take some time, but we can find a way—to make sure that
our children have health care.

This was an accurate outline of the Clinton administration's
health policy agenda for the next four years, and that agenda was a
success with a Republican Congress. Indeed, in the final two years of
his administration, with a sizable part of this agenda achieved at least
nominally in new legislation, Clinton could move on to new health
policy issues (particularly the "patients' bill of rights"). But what
made these initiatives so politically attractive to the Clinton administration and ultimately to many Republicans was not that they were
"step-by-step" proposals as such but that they targeted coverage at
people without insurance without doing anything to change the coverage that insured people already have. Americans have generally
offered majority or near-majority support for tax increases to pay
for increased health coverage of the uninsured in polls (at least in
principle—as this paper has demonstrated, they take little interest in
those programs for the uninsured that already exist).[29] What polls
made blatant during the Clinton health reform debate, however, is
that most insured Americans did not want to give up their employer
coverage in favor of public coverage, and they were easily convinced
to oppose a proposal that appeared to do that.[30]

That is even more true today, and erstwhile staunch supporters
of more universal public coverage are increasingly abandoning that
goal. Ron Pollack, head of the prominent liberal health policy lobby
Families USA, is a longtime advocate of national public health insurance. Nevertheless, as mentioned earlier in this report, he has recently thrown his support to a much more incremental set of reforms, a
combination of Medicaid and CHIP expansion to parents and childless adults and refundable tax credits to purchase private insurance
that is a joint proposal with the Health Insurance Association of
America (HIAA), a major health insurers' lobby, and the American
Hospital Association. His reasoning for this change of tactics, in
an article cowritten with Charles Kahn of HIAA, is notable for its
directness: "Simply stated, if asked to make a change that affects
their own health coverage, many of those who are insured will not

support reform efforts. This means that any proposal that changes the form of people's health coverage, appears to diminish the scope or quality of that coverage, or threatens to result in increased costs for that coverage is likely to provoke unbeatable opposition."[31]

But any effort to give blanket public coverage to all of the uninsured would inevitably involve some displacement of private coverage as well, opening the plan to charges of a government takeover of health care. That is because there is no way to focus public health coverage on those without insurance as such: it is virtually impossible to distinguish directly between those who cannot access or afford employer coverage and those who find it cheaper to turn down or drop available employer coverage and sign up for government coverage instead. Basing eligibility for public coverage for the nonelderly on income is a legacy of Medicaid's ties to welfare, but it is also a straightforward way to target a lot of uninsured people without significantly disturbing the private coverage of the majority of Americans. Yet, as described earlier, the typical results of means testing—the hassles to verify income and the periodic spells of eligibility for many beneficiaries—may in and of themselves be a major barrier to enrollment. Furthermore, programs designed for low-income people have trouble attracting working people and retirees, and they lack the political strength of programs that help wealthier citizens, particularly in the majority of states in which health care programs are off the radar screen of public opinion.

4

RETHINKING THE MODEL FROM THE GROUND UP

At several points this report has compared Medicaid and related programs to Medicare, comparisons that put the former in a distinctly unflattering light: Medicare covered its entire target population quickly, while Medicaid, CHIP, QMB/SLMB, and state drug programs have faced initial delays in state adoption and ongoing under-enrollment problems; almost every physician in America takes Medicare patients, while in many states Medicaid enrollees have much more limited access to physician's offices; Medicare is politically strong both in terms of interest group politics and public opinion, whereas state-administered health programs are marginal in local politics, marginal enough that at repeated intervals state governments have been able to contrive openly to prevent eligible people from enrolling. These comparisons all point to a program more like Medicare—national, centralized, and universal health coverage—as an alternative to Medicaid.

Medicare expansion is an approach that many liberal Democrats took in the House when the Clinton health reform bill was on its doomed legislative voyage. The main problem with that approach is that it could not come close to passage in today's political environment. Indeed, it is remarkable that Medicare got passed at all. That only happened because of the extraordinary circumstances of the election landslide of 1964. Medicare was held up all through the 1950s and early 1960s by the effective veto power of senior southern congressmen opposed to a big new federal program. But thanks to the Kennedy assassination and the nomination by Republicans of conservative Barry Goldwater, the 89th Congress of 1965–66 had an extremely large Democratic majority, by

American standards, of 68 to 32 in the Senate and 295 to 140 in the House, at a time when popular attitudes toward government were also much more positive than they are today. A context that liberal is unlikely to reappear any time soon.

More broadly, there is a trade-off in seeking more comprehensive solutions that are also less realistic politically. Many of those interested in health coverage expansions have been far too timid in thinking about that trade-off since 1994, but it must be considered. Chapter 3 laid out both the problems with the Medicaid model and the reasons expansions of the model have such political appeal inside the Beltway. The challenge in fixing existing programs and planning new or extended coverage is to keep the political strengths—that is, to keep frontline administration out of Washington and to avoid the appearance of threatening employer coverage—while dealing with the underlying problems.

Below, organized around the five basic problems with the Medicaid model described in the previous chapter, are some alternative structures for public coverage to replace Medicaid as we know it.

PROBLEM 2:
MEANS TESTING MAKES IT HARD TO ENROLL PEOPLE BECAUSE OF PAPERWORK TO VERIFY ELIGIBILITY INITIALLY AND AT REPEATED INTERVALS

Solution: Change the Structure of Means-tested Health Insurance Programs to Enroll People Automatically and Verify Eligibility Retrospectively

The following statistic captures the problem with enrollment in Medicaid and similar programs: 84 percent of workers with children who can get family coverage from their employer sign up for it, while 45 percent of parents whose children are eligible for Medicaid and CHIP sign up for it.[1] This huge discrepancy has multiple causes, but the relative ease with which one can get employer insurance is one of the most important. In fact, a significantly higher percentage of low-income parents sign up for available employer coverage than enroll in Medicaid and CHIP when they are eligible, 64 percent versus 42 percent, even though employer coverage is usually a lot less affordable for poorer people.[2] Medicare, which makes enrollment almost automatic for people on Social Security, reaches virtually everyone eligible.

So one way to boost participation rates in Medicaid and similar programs, especially for people in good health, is to make enrollment as automatic as possible.[3] Some states have already taken steps in this direction, particularly in enrolling children. The most common simplifications have been to drop asset tests, allow off-site enrollment or mail-in applications, and require a renewal application only once a year. Several states also now take advantage of a formal federal option to make child applicants for Medicaid and CHIP eligible for benefits as soon as they apply rather than waiting for their documents to go through the verification process first.[4] Four states that monitored their "presumptive eligibility" programs found low rates of later denials of eligibility.[5]

But these represent limited progress when compared to enrollment in an employer plan or Medicare. Public programs still require applicants to document their income and to send in new documentation once a year (or even present it in person in many states).

A small number of states have taken somewhat bolder steps to make signing up for public coverage more like enrollment for employer coverage. A few states use online databases for birth and citizenship information instead of requiring applicants to get the documentation themselves. Seven states use "self-declaration" of income in their CHIP programs, an official term for letting people claim income eligibility without requiring documentary proof.[6] States then check the application information against tax records and other existing databases. Georgia, one of these seven states, makes reenrollment in CHIP even more hassle-free: it sends a letter to enrollees with the previous eligibility information and gives a telephone number to call if there are any changes; it has had strong levels of participation in CHIP.[7] Those states that allow self-certification have reported no increase in error or fraud rates as a result.[8] The federal Medicaid office confirmed in a September 2000 letter to state Medicaid quality control directors that self-declaration and other existing simplification measures have not caused any increase in erroneous or fraudulent enrollment.[9]

The experience of states with computer databases opens up the potential for truly automatic eligibility verification, particularly since all states are already federally required to conduct a computer check of their Medicaid and related health programs, to verify income, and to look at a random sample of cases for quality and fraud control. States could enroll people without any documentation and then check income tax records, citizenship records, or employer insurance records (all records that states are already cross-matching for a portion of enrollees). States could require documentation after the fact for those whose eligibility is called into question, and they could follow up by seeking reimbursement and penalties for those found ineligible.

As noted above, those states that have implemented partly automatic enrollment have had no noticeable fraud problems despite dropping documentation requirements. But going further toward truly automatic enrollment would almost certainly allow for some people to get benefits who were not eligible. Experience so far indicates that it would not be many, and those could be identified and tracked with existing databases and possibly prosecuted. Moreover, right now the underenrollment problem is multiple orders of magnitude greater than the problem of fraudulent enrollment. When half of those eligible for public coverage or more are going without health insurance, there is good reason to shift from a welfare-oriented, fraud-prevention enrollment model to one that puts a higher priority on signing people up and reducing the numbers going without insurance.

As we have seen, signing up those who express an interest in enrolling is only half the battle. Many working people and retirees are unaware that they are eligible for public health coverage. Here again the demographic and income information available on government databases could accommodate a basic change in program operations. Several states use records from other means-tested programs—such as school lunches; the Women, Infants and Children program; and food stamps—to simplify enrollment. A couple of states have gone further by targeting mailings toward enrollees in other means-tested programs. South Carolina, Connecticut, and Rhode Island, three states with strong CHIP enrollment relative to need, conducted broad mailings concerning CHIP based on income as reported in tax records (Connecticut) or school registration (Rhode Island and South Carolina).[10]

Combining these approaches would make public program enrollment a lot more like signing up for employer coverage. The federal government would mandate that states: (1) mail applications to broad categories of residents likely to be eligible; (2) allow those likely "eligibles" to enroll just by checking off their eligibility in a simple application; (3) verify eligibility in state audits using the same computerized databases that they already use to double-check Medicaid eligibility for a sample of enrollees. If signing up were that easy, a lot more people would be insured.

PROBLEM 1: WORKING PEOPLE AND RETIREES ARE NOT AWARE OF OR COMFORTABLE WITH "WELFARE" HEALTH PROGRAMS;

PROBLEM 3: PROGRAMS WITHOUT BENEFITS TO THE MIDDLE CLASS ARE POLITICALLY WEAK IN INTEREST GROUP POLITICS;

PROBLEM 4: HEALTH PROGRAMS ARE MARGINAL IN STATE ELECTORAL POLITICS

Solution: Broaden the Reach of State-administered Programs to Include Portions of the Middle Class who Cannot Get Health Insurance

While 83 percent of adults describe Medicare as "somewhat" or "very important to them personally in terms of how much they currently benefit from it or expect to benefit from it," only 49 percent of adults even describe themselves as "somewhat familiar" or more so with Medicaid (and presumably quite a bit fewer would assert that it is important to them because they expect to benefit from it).[11] This goes a long way toward explaining why Medicaid model programs cannot reach many working people (who do not think they are eligible), and it is a major reason for the irrelevancy of these programs in interest group politics and in public opinion as well.

Yet more than 57 percent of all *insured* adults polled in 2000 worried that they might not be able to afford health care that they need, and 47 percent worried about losing health insurance and missing out on needed preventive care.[12] Voters are concerned about losing health insurance and needing health care they cannot pay for, then, but they do not look to Medicaid for help. By and large they are right because, unless they are on welfare or they want coverage for their children, they cannot get it.

Medicaid and its policy cousins are open to the following groups of people: children; no-income or very low-income parents; very low-income elderly; and adults so disabled that the government determines that they cannot work. These groups are all eligible for welfare, and this list is a legacy of Medicaid's connection to welfare. When the Medicaid model has tried to reach beyond welfare and the very poor within these populations—children's coverage up to 200 percent of poverty, or Medicare cost-sharing support in the QMB/SLMB program, or state prescription drug programs for the elderly—a lot of those eligible have not been aware of it. If the goal is to start enrolling uninsured working people and underinsured retirees and additionally to raise the political profile of health insurance programs outside of Medicare, it is imperative to break the welfare-Medicaid connection decisively.

One compelling way to do this is by reaching those in the middle class who cannot get health insurance. There are two groups of working-age adults who have particularly acute needs for health insurance but poor access to it, and they are left out of the current system of public coverage: people who are not deemed wholly disabled but have major disabilities that make it hard for them to find full-time jobs with benefits and people with serious, long-term health problems. Basing health coverage eligibility on the old welfare standard leaves them out.

Employer-sponsored health coverage often excludes bad health risks, people with low incomes, and people in part-time jobs. More specifically, it excludes people with physical or mental disabilities who can work but cannot work in a full-time job and therefore do not get health benefits. Employer coverage also leaves out those with chronic conditions and illnesses that are expensive to treat but do not limit or only partly limit their ability to work, who must hope they find employment at a big firm that can spread individual health costs across a large number of covered employees. If people with serious health problems do not get such a job, then the individual and small-employer health insurance markets are inaccessible to them in ways that are difficult to resolve through market regulation. They are likely either to get rejected outright by insurers, to face extraordinarily high premiums, or to get coverage that excludes payment for their illness.

To reach the first group—those with functional disabilities who can and should work but whose disability puts them at risk for lack of access to jobs with benefits—an incremental change will go a long way. The current standard for disabled adults can be loosened to include not only those who cannot work at all but also those whose disability means that their work capacity is seriously compromised.

In order to reach those with chronic illnesses, however, to focus on employability at all is to miss the target: their claim on public coverage stems from the urgency of their health needs and their unattractiveness to private insurers. A substantial number of states have tried (and generally failed) to get broad coverage to chronically ill adults by setting up special, high-risk private insurance pools that typically become extraordinarily expensive and fail to enroll many. Another alternative, an "employer mandate," also is fraught with problems. Any effort simply to require small or part-time employers to cover employees by way of private insurance markets could lead to unemployment and job discrimination against those considered poor health risks; the cost of coverage for people with serious health problems in low-income jobs may be larger than the rest of their compensation package. An employer mandate would meet the same fierce opposition of the small-business community that posed a great political obstacle to the original Clinton health care reform plan. A number of states have tried to subsidize employers or employees directly to help pay for health coverage. These programs have all been small, ranging from several hundred to several thousand enrollees in ten states in 2000.[13] They have found that, without almost total subsidy, most employees and small employers will not buy in, while state governments rightly fear that such larger subsidies would encourage employers currently paying for coverage themselves to take advantage of the public system and thereby defeat the purpose of routing taxpayer support through employer coverage.

That leaves direct public coverage. So far, only Tennessee has opened public coverage to people with serious health problems by including "uninsurables"—which the state defines broadly as adults who have been turned down at least once for private insurance because of a health condition—as an eligibility group in its Medicaid expansion, called TennCare. Although this is by definition one of the most expensive groups of people to cover, it also has been one

of the most stable beneficiary categories through TennCare's tur-
bulent first few years, one of the only expanded eligibility types for
which the state has not yet felt the need to close off new enrollment. Nevertheless, Tennessee's governor recently endorsed an official commission's recommendation that TennCare eliminate
coverage for many of these "uninsurable" adults, arguing that an
independent medical screening could weed out the substantial number of them that could actually get coverage either from their
employer or in the individual insurance market. Critics have aired
vehement concerns that the cutback would deny coverage to people
who need health care desperately. With 2002 a gubernatorial election year in Tennessee, the debate over this proposed retrenching is
a major test of the political durability of public coverage for the
"uninsurable" through Medicaid.

However that debate turns out, by covering so many low-
income or ill adults outside of the welfare system—a quarter of the
state's population—Tennessee has markedly increased the saliency of
health programs in state politics. And no one talks about underenrollment in Tennessee. The state apparently avoided the drop-off
in enrollment that accompanied welfare reform in so many states
precisely because TennCare is no longer a welfare program, as a
major study observed: "Although the number of Tennessee residents qualifying for welfare benefits declined 45 percent from
January 1994 (when TennCare was implemented) to June 1997,
from 303,000 to 167,000, enrollment in Medicaid decreased only
slightly during this period. One possible explanation for stability in
Medicaid enrollment despite the effects of welfare reform is
TennCare's separate identity. Because of the large size of the
TennCare program and its inclusion of non-Medicaid eligible residents, it is less likely to be identified with state welfare programs."[14]

An eligibility standard based on urgency of health needs and
unattractiveness of potential clients to private insurers must balance the need to cover the people who cannot pay for desperately
needed care against the risk of turning public coverage into an all-
purpose dumping ground for people who get sick. TennCare's existing, simple "prior denial of coverage" standard has clearly risked
the latter, which is part of the rationale for Governor Sundquist's
proposed cutbacks. But for all its problems (low reimbursement
levels, failed insurers, broad state budgetary weakness, and high
turnover of program administrators, among others) TennCare has

been successful at maintaining meaningful health coverage for large numbers of otherwise uninsurable people. TennCare has been controversial, both because of its administrative failures and because it is an expansive government program in an increasingly conservative, low-tax state. But when it comes to new thinking on eligibility, TennCare's fundamental political strength and enrollment success—even in light of the governor's recent proposal—ought to be an impressive and encouraging example.

PROBLEM 5: POORER STATES FACE INTENSE FISCAL PRESSURE, YET THEY HAVE THE GREATEST NEED

Solution: Shift More of the Funding Responsibility for Means-tested Health Insurance Programs to the Federal Government

As discussed in Chapter 3, poor states have strict eligibility criteria and low expenditures in their Medicaid programs relative to need—they have more uninsured people and less money to cover them with. The primary tool used in the Medicaid model for dealing with this disparity is a formula that varies the federal "match rate" for state expenditures—the percentage of total state Medicaid expenditures actually paid by the federal government. That rate varies from 50 percent to 78 percent for Medicaid based on state per capita income, so that wealthy states see Medicaid expenses matched dollar for dollar, while the poorest states get about three and a half dollars for every one that they spend. One criticism of the formula is that it is unfair to jurisdictions that are wealthy on average but have a lot of rich and poor people alike, such as Washington, D.C., California, and New York. Of still greater concern, this formula is manifestly not enough to compensate for the double fiscal jeopardy of more limited resources and greater need in poorer states, hence the huge disparities in how much state programs spend relative to the actual insurance needs of their populations that were previously identified in this report.

The most direct way to avoid the inequities of state variations in coverage would be to nationalize these programs. But keeping bureaucratic administration in the states is politically sacrosanct in Washington. Nationalizing and evening out funding need not mean centralizing administration, though. One option is simply to increase the match rates. CHIP expenditures are matched at the Medicaid rate plus 15 percent, giving the poorest states a six-to-one federal subsidy after adjustments. CHIP also shows that it is dangerous to apply such enhanced rates selectively. The difference between Medicaid and CHIP match rates led many states to enroll Medicaid-eligible children into CHIP, and in some states (like Idaho, as seen earlier) the lower Medicaid match rate still inhibited CHIP outreach efforts as many Medicaid-eligible children were discovered and enrolled along the way, straining budgets.

A second option is to select major aspects of state underperformance for enhanced match rates, particularly enrollment and reimbursement of primary care. States with high program enrollments relative to need (taking into account per capita state income and existing levels of private coverage) would receive a higher match rate, and primary care reimbursement would receive an enhanced rate across the board. Incentivizing in this way would make sure that practices contributing to underenrollment save less money and would reduce the temptation to extract budgetary savings from undercompensation of health care providers.

A more dramatic move to take the fiscal burden off of states could be the setting of a single, high, across-the-board national match rate: one precedent is the ninety-to-ten national match that was offered for states to upgrade Medicaid data reporting to meet a new standard in the 1980s. Note that this approach would offer an even greater increase in reimbursement to rich states than to poor ones, however.

Finally, the most sweeping nationalization would combine total federal funding with state administration. An example of this arrangement is the Supplementary Security Income (SSI) program that delivers cash benefits to poorest elderly and disabled. States run the program, while it is funded and supervised by the federal Social Security Administration, and many states supplement the federal cash benefit with their own money. (SSI also differs from Medicaid in its closer federal oversight of states and nationally uniform set of eligibility groups.) Full federal funding would remove virtually all of the pressure on states to limit enrollment and hold down reimbursement rates, and it would shift debates over eligibility and spending to Washington, where health programs are politically stronger and where the fiscal difficulties faced by poor states are irrelevant. Furthermore, SSI has had a strong record of enrollment success, with between 80 percent and 90 percent of eligible people with work disabilities participating. Nevertheless, while SSI offers a political precedent for splitting funding from administration, it is far from a full blueprint. Health coverage programs would have more complicated administrative power-sharing issues than SSI, as SSI does not deliver services but primarily determines eligibility and mails checks. And nationalizing funding would shift tens of billions of dollars of state costs to the federal government, something politically difficult in Washington under most circumstances (though naturally it would be politically popular in all state capitals, still more so in a time of renewed budget deficits.)

In any event, further federalization of Medicaid costs is opposed by the Bush administration, as became clear over the summer of 2001. In June, the National Governors Association (NGA) made a Medicaid proposal somewhat along the lines of the second option above—they outlined an enhanced federal match rate for all Medicaid coverage that is optional, meaning coverage above the minimum federal requirements that states need to satisfy for participation in Medicaid. The enhanced match rate would be the same as that now used for CHIP, which is the Medicaid rate plus an extra 15 percent, meaning a federal contribution of 65–85 percent of total spending, depending on state per capita income. All states already cover a lot of optional services and some or many people beyond those in categories mandated by law, so the higher match would shift a substantial portion of Medicaid expenses to the federal government, particularly for long-term care of the elderly. As the NGA emphasized, it also would reduce the costs to states of expanding Medicaid to new beneficiaries. The governors proposed to reduce Medicaid costs further by allowing states to cut part of their standard Medicaid service package to beneficiaries who fall outside classification as populations that must be covered and by allowing premiums and copayments for such beneficiaries or for optional services, all of which they cannot do now without a special waiver of Medicaid rules from the federal government.

The Bush administration, later in the summer of 2001, endorsed some parts of this proposal but not the enhanced match rate. The administration found acceptable provisions for states to reduce optional services and to introduce or increase cost sharing by participants; additionally, it made a federal commitment to sign off quickly on extending Medicaid to new populations, using these off-setting cuts for financing.

Both of these proposals have generated a good deal of criticism from advocates, who in particular fear the loss of benefits like prescription drugs and eye care for poor parents and senior citizens and the loss of special services for those with disabilities and mental illnesses, all of whom often qualify for Medicaid as beneficiaries even though federal law does not require them to be covered. But the key dispute is still that of who pays for Medicaid. The governors sought a major federalization of Medicaid financing, nominally in order to expand coverage to new populations. The administration refused to assume a higher share of Medicaid costs and instead established a greatly streamlined procedure for states to finance the spreading of Medicaid coverage by cutting back on benefits to existing enrollees, something that was always possible but had previously required long negotiations with the federal government. The governors' proposal would have eased some of the problems associated with partial financing of Medicaid by the states, but the Bush administration appears committed to the current structure and even to intensifying the capacity for (and therefore the pressure on) poor states to make cuts in the program. But if the inequities of Medicaid financing are going to be fixed, the federal government will have to assume more of the fiscal burden.

Conclusion

The alternatives laid out above are broad in scope. They are substantial departures from the current Medicaid model. But American health policy needs to turn off the incrementalist autopilot that Bill Clinton engaged in his 1995 State of the Union address. There is a great deal of room for reform beyond the blind expansion of the Medicaid model that has occupied us on and off since 1965 and especially recently, reform that can still avoid the political fears aroused by the concept of national health insurance. The bottom line is that the expansions of the past fifteen years are not getting us any closer to universal coverage. We need to think through more carefully a politically realistic approach that will succeed where the Medicaid model has failed.

NOTES

CHAPTER 1

1. Edward Kennedy and Orrin Hatch, "Health Insurance for Every Child," *Washington Post*, August 20, 1997, p. A25.

2. Government figures nominally showed a drop of about two million, but half of this was a statistical blip produced by a refinement in the way the Census Bureau asks about insurance coverage. Data available online from U.S. Department of Commerce, Bureau of the Census, http://www.census.gov/hhes/hlthins/historic/hihistt3.html, or search the Census Bureau site under "Health Insurance Historical Table 3."

CHAPTER 2

1. Theodore Marmor, *The Politics of Medicare*, 2d ed. (Hawthorne, N.Y.: Aldine de Gruyter, 2000), pp. 87–88.

2. Ibid., Chapter 2. See pp. 27–30 for the following paragraph.

3. Robert Stevens and Rosemary Stevens, *Welfare Medicine in America: A Case Study of Medicaid* (New York: Free Press, 1974), p. 33.

4. Diane Rowland, Alina Salganicoff, and Patricia Seliger Keenan, "The Key to the Door: Medicaid's Role in Improving Health Care for Women and Children," *Annual Review of Public Health* 20 (1999): 403–26; Karen Davis and Cathy Schoen, *Health and the War on Poverty: A Ten-Year Appraisal* (Washington, D.C.: Brookings Institution, 1978), pp. 62–67; Lisa Dubay and Genevieve M. Kenney, "Health Care Access and Use Among Low-Income Children: Who Fares Best?" *Health Affairs* 20, no. 1 (January/February 2001): 112–21.

5. See Rowland, Salganicoff, and Keenan, "Key to the Door," for a review of the substantial literature demonstrating this point.

6. John Holahan, "Restructuring Medicaid Financing: Implications of the NGA Proposal," Kaiser Commission on Medicaid and the Uninsured, Henry J. Kaiser Family Foundation, Washington, D.C., June 2001.

7. Davis and Schoen, *Health and the War on Poverty*, p. 56.

8. Ibid., pp. 56–62; Herbert Klarman, "Major Public Initiatives in Health Care," in Eli Ginzberg and Robert M. Solow, eds., *The Great Society* (New York: Basic Books 1974), p. 114.

9. Jon Gruber, John Kim, and Dina Mayzlin, "Physician Fees and Procedure Intensity," *Journal of Health Economics* 18, no. 4 (August 1999): 473–90.

10. In 1970, thirty states enrolled less than 50 percent of poor children in Medicaid, and only New York and California enrolled all poor children. See Karen Davis, *National Health Insurance: Benefits, Costs, and Consequences* (Washington, D.C.: Brookings Institution, 1975), pp. 48–49. Indeed, New York was a strong exception to many of the generalizations here. New York initially defined eligibility for its Medicaid program so broadly that Congress passed legislation to rein in the state in 1967. New York also runs an unusually large and generous Medicaid program, was the first state to enroll large numbers of children in working poor families into a CHIP-like program, and still runs an extraordinarily large CHIP program.

11. Davis and Schoen, *Health and the War on Poverty*, p. 59.

12. Ibid., p. 84.

13. Davis, *National Health Insurance*, p. 41.

14. For the latter figure, see James Morone, "American Political Culture and the Search for Lessons from Abroad," *Journal of Health Politics, Policy and Law* 15, no. 1 (Spring 1990): 128–43.

15. For Medicaid underenrollment, see Thomas M. Selden, Jessica S. Banthin, and Joel W. Cohen, "Medicaid's Problem Children: Eligible but not Enrolled," *Health Affairs* 17, no. 3 (May/June 1998): 192–200. For underenrollment figures for other means-tested programs, see, e.g., Rebecca M. Blank and Patricia Ruggles, "When Do Women Use Aid to Families with Dependent Children and Food Stamps? The Dynamics of Eligibility versus Participation," *Journal of Human Resources* 31, no. 1 (Winter 1996): 57–89.

16. Both of the above quotes are cited in Frank J. Thompson, "The Faces of Devolution," in Frank J. Thompson and John J. DiIulio, Jr., eds., *Medicaid and Devolution: A View from the States* (Washington, D.C.: Brookings Institution Press, 1998), p. 21.

17. Donald J. Boyd, *"Medicaid Devolution: A Fiscal Perspective,"* in ibid.

18. "Medicaid Enrollment in 50 States: June 1997 to December 1999," report prepared by Eileen R. Ellis, Vernon K. Smith, and David M. Rousseau,

Kaiser Commission on Medicaid and the Uninsured, Henry J. Kaiser Family Foundation, Washington, D.C., October 2000.

19. Karl Kronebusch, "Medicaid for Children: Federal Mandates, Welfare Reform, and Policy Backsliding," *Health Affairs* 20, no. 1 (January/February 2001): 97–111.

20. Bowen Garrett and John Holahan, "Health Insurance Coverage after Welfare," *Health Affairs* 19, no. 1 (January/February 2000): 175–84.

21. Kronebusch, "Medicaid for Children." Both South Carolina and Indiana were states with strong legislative and administrative support for child health coverage, and they were early leaders in CHIP enrollment as well.

22. Paul Offner, *Medicaid and the States* (New York: The Century Foundation Press, 1999), p. 16.

23. American Dental Association, "Report of the Aim for Change in Medicaid Conference," 1999, available online at www.ADA.org.

24. Stephen Norton and Stephen Zuckerman, "Trends in Medicaid Physician Fees, 1993–1998," *Health Affairs* 19, no. 4 (July/August 2000): 222–32

25. Offner, *Medicaid and the States, p. 17.*

26. *Physician Socioeconomic Statistics, 2000–2002,* Center for Health Policy Research, American Medical Association, Chicago, 2002, Table 43.

27. John Billings, Nina Parikh, and Tod Mijanovich, "Emergency Room Use: The New York Story," Issue Brief no. 434, Commonwealth Fund, New York, November 2000.

28. John Holahan and Len Nichols, "State Health Policy in the 1990s," in Robert F. Rich and William D. White, eds., *Health Policy, Federalism and the American States* (Washington, D.C.: Urban Institute, 1996); my analysis here draws more broadly on Bruce Vladeck, "Medicaid Managed Care: Goals, Accomplishments and Prospects," speech delivered at "Medicaid Managed Care: A Vision Revisited," United Hospital Fund conference, New York, July 11, 2001.

29. Marsha Lillie-Blanton and Barbara Lyons, "Managed Care and Low-Income Populations: Recent State Experiences," *Health Affairs* 17, no. 3 (May/June 1998): 238–47; Stephen Zuckerman and Niall Brennan, "Medicaid Managed Care and Beneficiary Access and Use," unpublished paper presented at an Urban Institute conference, Washington, D.C., 2000, available from the authors on request; Douglas R. Wholey, Lawton R. Burns, and Risa Lavizzo-Mourey, "Managed Care and the Delivery of Primary Care to the Elderly and the Chronically Ill," *Health Services Research* 33, no. 2 (June 1998): 322–53; Janet B. Mitchell, Galina Khatutsky, and Nancy L.

Swigonski, "Impact of the Oregon Health Plan on Children with Special Health Care Needs," *Pediatrics* 107, no. 4 (April 2001): 736–43; John Ware et al., "Differences in 4 Year Health Outcomes for Elderly and Poor, Chronically Ill Patients Treated in HMO and Fee for Service Systems," *Journal of the American Medical Association* 276, no. 13 (October 2, 1996): 1039–47.

30. John Holahan, Suresh Rangarajan, and Matthew Schirmer, "Medicaid Managed Care Payment Rates in 1998," *Health Affairs* 18, no. 3 (May/June 1999): 217–27.

31. Ibid.

32. Suzanne Felt-Lisk, "The Changing Medicaid Managed Care Market: Trends in Commercial Plans' Participation," Kaiser Commission on Medicaid and the Uninsured, Henry J. Kaiser Family Foundation, Washington, D.C., May 1999.

33. The mandatory buy-in was part of the ill-fated Medicare Catastrophic Coverage Act (MCCA). When combined with some of the other changes in MCCA, the new costs to states from the QMB program were supposed to be more than fully offset by savings from Medicare expansions. Those savings did not materialize beyond the first year because MCCA was repealed in 1989. See Marilyn Moon, Niall Brennan, and Misha Segal, "Options for Aiding Low-Income Medicare Beneficiaries," *Inquiry* 35, no. 3 (Fall 1998): 346–56.

34. Because of the way HCFA and the states report QMB enrollment, statistics on QMB can lump together beneficiaries who are eligible for full Medicaid and those participating in the QMB program alone. Therefore different modeling techniques produce varying statistics on enrollment. The General Accounting Office found just 2.4 million QMB-only enrollees in 1998 and a similar number in 1995 ("Low Income Medicare Beneficiaries," GAO/HEHS-99-61, U.S. General Accounting Office, April 1999). But the Alliance for Health Reform estimated QMB enrollment at only 367,000 in 1995. (See Ellen O'Brien and Diane Rowland, "Medicare and Medicaid for the Elderly and Disabled Poor," Kaiser Commission on Medicaid and the Uninsured, Henry J. Kaiser Family Foundation, Washington, D.C., May 1999; "Managed Care and Vulnerable Americans: Medicare and Medicaid Dual Eligibles," Issue Brief no. 97–01, Alliance for Health Reform, Washington, D.C., March 1997.) Families USA ("Shortchanged: Billions Withheld from Medicare Beneficiaries," report no. 98–103, Families USA, Washington, D.C., July 1998) estimates QMB enrollment at 4–4.5 million, and Moon, Brennan, and Segal ("Options for Aiding Low-Income Medicare Beneficiaries") find similar figures pegging QMB enrollment at 78 percent of

those eligible, but these authors explicitly include those enrolled in full Medicaid and the Supplementary Security Income program in their QMB count. SLMB enrollment is more consistently counted at about 200,000, or 14–16 percent of eligibility.

35. Families USA, "Shortchanged"; "Variations in State Medicaid Buy-In Practices for Low-Income Medicare Beneficiaries: A 1999 Update," prepared by Patricia B. Nemore, Henry J. Kaiser Family Foundation, Washington, D.C., December 1999.

36. See Margo L. Rosenbach and JoAnn Lamphere, "Bridging the Gaps between Medicare and Medicaid: The Case of QMBs and SLMBs," report no. 9902, AARP Public Policy Institute, Washington, D.C., January 1999, for explanation of how estimates of more than 100 percent enrollment are possible.

37. "Variations in State Medicaid Buy-In Practices."

38. Peter Cunningham, "Targeting Communities with High Rates of Uninsured Children", *Health Affairs,* Web Exclusive, July 2001, pp. w20–w29, available online at http://130.94.25.113/readeragent.php?ID=/usr/local/apache/sites/healthaffairs.org/htdocs/Library/v20n5/s2.pdf; Lisa Dubay et al., "Children's Eligibility for Medicaid and SCHIP," Urban Institute, Washington, D.C., March 2000.

39. Robert Mills, "Health Insurance Coverage: 2000," *Current Population Reports,* U.S. Department of Commerce, Bureau of the Census, September 2001, 1988–98 data available online from the Census Bureau, search under "Health Insurance Historical Table 3." As explained in the Mills report, the Census Bureau changed its questionnaire in 2000 to correct a flaw that was leading to an overestimate of the number of uninsured of about 8 percent. This new format has been employed only for 1999 and 2000 surveys, however, meaning that all pre-1999 years include this 8 percent overestimate, while the past two years do not. To allow for comparisons between pre-1999 and post-1999 numbers, the Census Bureau provided estimates of the uninsured using the old methodology for 1999 and 2000 as well, and I have used those here. Using the new methodology, the percentage of children who are uninsured goes down to 12.6 percent in 1999 and 11.6 percent in 2000, and presumably it would have been about 1–1.5 percent lower for all the pre-1999 years as well. Note that the 23.2 percent figure for public coverage in 2000 would have been about 23.3 percent under the old methodology, while private coverage would have been 70.5 percent rather than 69.3 percent. Figure 2–4 on private and public coverage levels includes extrapolations of old methodology rates for 2000 provided to the author by the Bureau of the Census in a personal communication.

40. Dubay et al., "Children's Eligibility for Medicaid and SCHIP"; Margo Edmunds, Martha Teitelbaum, and Cassy Gleason, "All Over the Map: A Progress Report on the State Children's Health Insurance Program (CHIP)," Health Division, Children's Defense Fund, Washington, D.C., July 2000, estimates 2 million eligible but not enrolled using a then current estimate of 2 million CHIP enrollees.

41. Cunningham, "Targeting Communities with High Rates of Uninsured Children."

42. "CHIP Program Enrollment: December 2000," prepared by Vernon K. Smith, David M. Rousseau, and Jocelyn A. Guyer, Kaiser Commission on Medicaid and the Uninsured, Henry J. Kaiser Family Foundation, Washington, D.C., September 2001.

43. Ibid.; Alina Salganicoff, Patricia Seliger Keenan, and David Liska, "Child Health Facts: National and State Profiles of Coverage," Kaiser Commission on the Future of Medicaid, Henry J. Kaiser Family Foundation, Washington, D.C., January 1998.

44. "CHIP Program Enrollment: December 2000"; Salganicoff, Keenan, and Liska, "Child Health Facts."

45. "Making Child Health Coverage a Reality: Lessons from Case Studies of Medicaid and CHIP Outreach and Enrollment Strategies," prepared by Renee Schwalberg et al., Kaiser Commission on Medicaid and the Uninsured, Henry J. Kaiser Family Foundation, Washington, D.C., September 1999; Margo Rosenbach et al., "Implementation of the State Children's Health Insurance Program: Momentum Is Increasing After a Modest Start: First Annual Report," Mathematica Policy Research, Inc., Cambridge, Mass., January 2001; "Making It Simple: Medicaid for Children and CHIP Income Eligibility Guidelines and Enrollment Procedures: Findings from a 50-State Survey," prepared by Donna Cohen Ross and Laura Cox, Kaiser Commission on Medicaid and the Uninsured, Henry J. Kaiser Family Foundation, Washington, D.C., October 2000; Dawn Horner, Wendy Lazarus, and Beth Morrow, "Express Lane Eligibility: How to Enroll Large Groups of Eligible Children in Medicaid and CHIP," Kaiser Commission on Medicaid and the Uninsured, Henry J. Kaiser Family Foundation, Washington, D.C., December 1999; "Medicaid and Children: Overcoming Barriers to Enrollment: Findings from a National Survey," prepared by Michael Perry et al., Kaiser Commission on Medicaid and the Uninsured, Henry J. Kaiser Family Foundation, Washington, D.C., January 2000; Dennis Andrulis, Tamar Bauer, and Sarah Hopkins, "Strategies to Increase Enrollment in Children's Health Insurance Programs: A Guide to Outreach, Marketing and Enrollment in New York and Other States," New York

Forum for Child Health, New York Academy of Medicine, New York, January 1999; Deborah Bachrach et al., "Closing Coverage Gaps: Improving Retention Rates in New York's Medicaid and Child Health Plus Programs," report, New York State Coalition of PHSPs, New York, December 2000.

46. "In the past, many eligibility workers focused on moving people off welfare and Medicaid. . . . Now, the orientation in most state SCHIP programs is that staff should encourage and assist eligible families during both the application and redetermination processes." Rosenbach et al., "Implementation of the State Children's Health Insurance Program."

47. Ian Hill, "Charting New Courses for Children's Health Insurance," *Policy and Practice* 58, no. 4 (December 2000): 30–38.

48 "Medicaid and SCHIP: Comparisons of Outreach, Enrollment Practices, and Benefits," GAO/HEHS-00-86, U.S. General Accounting Office, April 2000, p. 30.

49. David Gross and Sharon Bee, "State Pharmacy Assistance Programs," report no. 9905, AARP Public Policy Institute, Washington, D.C., April 1999.

50. "State Pharmacy Programs," GAO/HEHS-00-162, U.S. General Accounting Office, September 2000.

51. Marilyn W. Serafini, "Prescription Drugs: The State Experience," *National Journal,* October 7, 2000, pp. 3/74–3/75.

52. "EPIC Evaluation Report to the Governor and Legislature", EPIC [Elderly Pharmaceutical Insurance Coverage] Advisory Committee, State of New York, 1996, p. 31.

CHAPTER 3

1. See, for example, Rowland, Salganicoff, and Keenan, "Key to the Door"; "Health Coverage Update: Children's Health Insurance," Issue Brief no. 00–01, Alliance for Health Reform, Washington, D.C., March 2000; Mary Jo O'Brien et al., "State Experiences with Access Issues under Children's Health Insurance Expansions," pub. no. 384, Commonwealth Fund, New York, May 2000; Serafini, "Prescription Drugs"; Heidi Shaner, "Dual Eligible Outreach and Enrollment: A View from the States," Health Care Financing Administration, March 1999, available online at http://www.hcfa.gov/medicaid/dualelig/o&erpt.htm.

2. Covering Kids Initiative report, Robert Wood Johnson Foundation, Princeton, N.J., August 9, 2000; cf. "Medicaid and Children: Overcoming Barriers to Enrollment."

3. "Medicaid and Children: Overcoming Barriers to Enrollment," Figure 6.

4. "Health Care Reform: Potential Difficulties in Determining Eligibility for Low-Income People," GAO/HEHS-94-176, U.S. General Accounting Office, July 11, 1994.

5. "Medicare Facts and Faces: Making Health Care Affordable for People with Low Incomes," policy brief, Medicare Rights Center, New York, Fall 2000.

6. "Variations in State Medicaid Buy-In Practices."

7. Jennifer Weiss, "Real Access? An Investigative Report on Access to the Medicare Savings Programs for People with Medicare in New York City," Medicare Rights Center, New York, August 2001.

8. For this and the other statistics cited here, see "Making It Simple."

9. Paul Peterson has argued in two books that many states will inevitably underfund redistributive programs for fear of attracting poorer populations. Paul E. Peterson, Barry G. Rabe, and Kenneth K. Wong, *When Federalism Works* (Washington, D.C.: Brookings Institution, 1986); Paul E. Peterson, *The Price of Federalism* (Washington, D.C.: Brookings Institution, 1995). Paul Offner maintains that a dramatic scaling back of state responsibilities in Medicaid will give clearer division of accountability for the program between the states and the federal government (Offner, *Medicaid and the States*).

10. Christopher Trenholm and Susanna King, *Disparities in State Health Coverage: A Matter of Policy or Fortune?* Academy for Health Services Research and Health Policy, Washington, D.C., December 2000.

11. Rosenbach and Lamphere, "Bridging the Gaps between Medicare and Medicaid."

12. For California governor Gray Davis's veto remarks, see "Two Health-Care Access Bills Vetoed: Gov. Gray Davis Says the State Can't Afford the Additional Spending," *Sacramento Bee*, October 10, 2001.

13. CNN/Voter News Service exit poll.

14. Personal communication from Voter News Service, and wire service reports.

15. Steven Gold, "Health Care and the Fiscal Crisis of the States," in Rich and White, *Health Policy, Federalism and the American States*.

16. Boyd, "Medicaid Devolution," pp. 81–85; Trenholm and King, *Disparities in State Health Coverage*.

17. Trenholm and King, *Disparities in State Health Coverage*.

18. Ibid., Table 5.

19. Pamela A. Paul-Shaheen, "The States and Health Care Reform: The Road Traveled and Lessons Learned from Seven that Took the Lead,"

Journal of Health Politics, Policy and Law 23, no. 2 (April 1998): 319–61; Penelope Lemov, "Critical Condition," *Governing*, October 1999, pp. 22–27.

20. "Without exception, the key 'crisis' that served as the rallying cry for comprehensive state reform in these seven states was escalating health care costs. Those advocating for reform found early on that framing the issue as a cost 'crisis'—for the middle class, the government and/or the business community—significantly increased the likelihood that political inertia could be overcome and policy action advanced." Paul-Shaheen, "States and Health Care Reform."

21. Jeremy Alberga et al., *State of the States Report,* Academy for Health Services Research and Health Policy, Washington, D.C., January 2001, p. 8.

22. "Health Insurance Coverage in America," report prepared by Catherine Hoffman and Mary Beth Pohl, Kaiser Commission on Medicaid and the Uninsured, Henry J. Kaiser Family Foundation, Washington, D.C., February 2002.

23. Christopher J. Conover and Hester H. Davies, "The Role of TennCare in Health Policy for Low-Income People in Tennessee," occasional paper no. OP-33 Urban Institute, Washington, D.C., February 2000; Anna Aizer et al., "Medicaid Managed Care and Low Income Populations: Four Years' Experience with TennCare," Kaiser/Commonwealth Low Income Project, May 1999.

24. "Health Insurance Status of Massachusetts Children," Access Update, no. 2, and "Health Insurance Status of Massachusetts Adults," Access Update, no. 3, Massachusetts Division of Health Care Finance and Policy, June 2001, available online at http://www.state.ma.us/dhcfp/pages/pdf/access4.pdf; Trenholm and King, *Disparities in State Health Coverage.*

25. Robert C. Lieberman, *Shifting the Color Line: Race and the American Welfare State* (Cambridge, Mass.: Harvard University Press, 1998); see also several of the essays in Margaret Weir, Ann Shola Orloff, and Theda Skocpol, eds., *The Politics of Social Policy in the United States* (Princeton, N.J.: Princeton University Press, 1988).

26. Bruce C. Vladeck, "The Political Economy of Medicare," *Health Affairs* 18, no. 1 (January/February 1999): 22–36.

27. "Opposites Attract, and Team Up on a Flood of Legislation," *Los Angeles Times,* May 8, 1997, p. A5.

28. *Congressional Record,* June 17, 1997.

29. See the periodic public opinion surveys sponsored by the Henry J. Kaiser Family Foundation and the Harvard School of Public Health, available online at www.kff.org.

30. Daniel Yankelovich, "The Debate that Wasn't: The Public and the Clinton Plan," *Health Affairs* 14, no. 1 (Spring 1995): 7–23.

31. Charles N. Kahn III and Ronald F. Pollack, "Building a Consensus for Expanding Health Coverage," *Health Affairs 20,* no. 1 (January/February 2001): 40–48.

CHAPTER 4

1. Cunningham, "Targeting Communities with High Rates of Uninsured Children."

2. Ibid.

3. I am indebted to Bruce C. Vladeck and Barbara Cooper for providing many of the specifics for these proposals.

4. "Making It Simple."

5. Andrulis, Bauer, and Hopkins, "Strategies to Increase Enrollment in Children's Health Insurance Programs."

6. Margo Rosenbach et al., "Implementation of the State Children's Health Insurance Program," first annual SCHIP report, Health Care Financing Administration, January 2001, p. 58.

7. "Making It Simple," p. 9. For Georgia's CHIP enrollment, see "CHIP Program Enrollment: December 2000."

8. Bachrach et al., "Closing Coverage Gaps"; Vicky Pulos and Lisa Gallin Lynch, "Outreach Strategies in the State Children's Health Insurance Program," Families USA, Washington, D.C., June 1998, p. 11.

9. "Letter to State Quality Control Directors," Center for Medicaid and State Operations, Health Care Financing Administration, September 12, 2000.

10. Pulos and Lynch, "Outreach Strategies in the State Children's Health Insurance Program," p. 11.

11. Survey results for Medicare: NBC News/Wall Street Journal Poll, December 1997; for Medicaid: Kaiser/NewsHour Survey, May 2000.

12. Kaiser/NewsHour Survey, May 2000.

13. Sharon Silow-Carroll, Stephanie E. Anthony, and Jack A. Meyer, "State and Local Initiatives to Enhance Health Coverage for the Working Uninsured," pub. no. 424, Commonwealth Fund, New York, November 2000.

14. Aizer et al., "Medicaid Managed Care and Low Income Populations," p. 21.

INDEX

Note: Page numbers followed by letters *f, n,* and *t* refer to figures, notes, and tables, respectively.

ABOUT THE AUTHOR

Eliot Fishman is currently senior research associate at the Institute for Medicare Practice, Mount Sinai School of Medicine, New York. He writes frequently on health care policy and Medicaid issues, and his writings have appeared in the *Washington Post*, *Health Affairs*, and other publications. He received a Ph.D. in political science from Yale University. He lives in Stamford, Connecticut, with his wife, Suzanne Wachsstock, and his sons, Joshua and Leor.